Manual of Stem Cell and Bone Marrow Transplantation

Over the past 35 years, stem cell and bone marrow transplantation have evolved from experimental therapies to well-established and widely used treatments for a variety of malignant and non-malignant conditions. This is a practical pocket manual for all members of the stem cell and bone marrow transplant team, based on a popular in-house handbook used at the Dana-Farber Cancer Institute. The manual covers all aspects of the transplantation process, from stem cell processing through management of transplant-related complications. Evaluation and counseling of patients and donors, preventative care, and conditioning regimens are also covered, making this an ideal resource for nurses as well. The text is handily arranged in outline format to maximize the usefulness and convenience of this resource.

Joseph H. Antin, MD, is Professor of Medicine at Harvard Medical School and Chief of the Stem Cell Transplantation Program at the Dana-Farber Brigham and Women's Cancer Center, Boston, Massachusetts.

Deborah Yolin Raley, MS, PA-C, is Chief Physician Assistant in the Hematopoietic Stem Cell Transplant Program at the Dana-Farber Cancer Institute, Boston, Massachusetts.

Manual of Stem Cell and Bone Marrow Transplantation

JOSEPH H. ANTIN

Dana-Farber Cancer Institute

DEBORAH YOLIN RALEY

Dana-Farber Cancer Institute

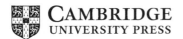

CAMBRIDGE UNIVERSITY PRESS

CAMBRIDGE UNIVERSITY PRESS
Cambridge, New York, Melbourne, Madrid, Cape Town, Singapore, São Paulo, Delhi

Cambridge University Press
32 Avenue of the Americas, New York, NY 10013-2473, USA

www.cambridge.org
Information on this title: www.cambridge.org/9780521699754

First published 2009

Printed in the United States of America

A catalog record for this publication is available from the British Library.

Library of Congress Cataloging in Publication data
Antin, Joseph H.
  Manual of stem cell and bone marrow transplantation / Joseph H.
Antin, Deborah Yolin Raley.
    p. ; cm.
  Includes index.
  ISBN 978-0-521-69975-4 (pbk.)
  1. Bone marrow – Transplantation.   2. Stem cells – Transplantation.   I. Raley,
Deborah Yolin.   II. Dana-Farber Cancer Institute.   III. Title.   IV. Title: Manual
of stem cell transplantation.
  [DNLM: 1. Stem Cell Transplantation.   2. Bone Marrow Transplantation.
QU 325 A631d 2009]
  RD123.5.A58 2009
  617.4′410592–dc22   2008045257

ISBN 978-0-521-69975-4 paperback

Contents

Acknowledgments

The authors would like to thank the following people for their contribution to this project:

Theona Arsenalt

Dr. Lindsay Baden

Bonnie J. Campbell BS, RPh

Cara Dejong MS, RD, LDN, CNSN

Dr. Vincent Ho

Dr. Richard Kaufman

David Kubiak PharmD, BCPS

Dr. Francisco Marty

Dr. Paul Richardson

Dr. Robert Soiffer

Manual of Stem Cell and Bone Marrow Transplantation

1. RATIONALE FOR TRANSPLANTATION

Hematopoietic stem cell transplantation (HSCT) has the potential to cure a variety of benign and hematologic diseases that may be incurable with conventional therapy. In its broadest form, HSCT consists of three parts: a conditioning phase, stem cell infusion, and for allogeneic procedures, a method for prophylaxis of graft-versus-host disease (GVHD). There are, however, many variations of this framework. Conditioning regimens include various combinations of chemotherapy, radiotherapy, and immunotherapeutic agents. All conditioning regimens must produce at least enough immunosuppression to prevent graft rejection; beyond this, they can vary considerably in intensity, ranging from high dose regimens that result in complete ablation of the patient's bone marrow to reduced intensity regimens that cause only mild myelosuppression. Stem cells can be obtained from bone marrow (BM), peripheral blood (PB), or umbilical cord blood (UCB). Finally, GVHD prophylaxis can be achieved through immunosuppressive medications or graft manipulation (in particular T-cell depletion). The choice of conditioning regimen, stem cell source, and GVHD prophylaxis regimens varies on the basis of patient and disease characteristics as well as donor availability. In the case of allogeneic HSCT for hematologic malignancies, one of the principal goals is to allow engraftment and development of a donor-derived immune system, that can effect an immunologic attack against the recipient lymphohematopoietic system, and in particular against the tumor cells. This graft-versus-tumor (GVT) effect is a fundamental and unique aspect of allogeneic HSCT. In autologous transplantation, the main goal is to provide an opportunity for hematologic recovery after the administration of high dose therapy.

Not surprisingly, the outcome of HSCT depends on many patient factors, such as age and comorbidities; disease factors, such as diagnosis, disease stage, and prior therapy; donor factors, including human leukocyte antigen (HLA) and gender match; and transplantation factors, including conditioning regimen, stem cell source, and GVHD prophylaxis. The following table lists estimates of long-term survival for some of the hematologic malignancies and marrow disorders for which transplantation is commonly performed.

Disease	Approximate 5 year DFS (%)
AML/ALL	25–75 CR1
	20–40 CR2
	5–20 Refractory
CML	50–80 Stable phase
	20–40 Accelerated phase
	5–15 Blast crisis
NHL/HD/CLL	20–60 Chemosensitive relapse
	10–25 Refractory disease
MDS	50–65 RA/RARS
	10–35 RAEB
Multiple myeloma	10–25
Aplastic anemia	40–85

AML, acute myeloid leukemia; ALL, acute lymphoblastic leukemia; CLL, chronic lymphocytic leukemia; CML, chronic myeloid leukemia; HD, Hodgkin disease; MDS, myelodysplastic syndrome; NHL, non–Hodgkin lymphoma; RA, refractory anemia; RAEB, refractory anemia with excess blasts; RARS refractory anemia with ringed sideroblasts.

2. TYPES OF TRANSPLANTATION

AUTOLOGOUS TRANSPLANTATION

Autologous stem cell transplantation (or stem cell rescue) allows the administration of high-dose chemotherapy or chemoradiotherapy and eliminates myelotoxicity as a dose-limiting complication.

- The stem cell source can be either mobilized peripheral blood stem cells or bone marrow.
- Autologous transplantation is commonly used for lymphomas and myeloma and less commonly for leukemia.
- Autologous transplantation is also used for testicular cancer.
- In patients with leukemia and lymphoma, there is considerable concern over the reinfusion of occult tumor cells along with the marrow or peripheral blood progenitors. Therefore, numerous attempts to purge tumor cells from the stem cells have been undertaken. However, it is unclear whether such manipulation affects relapse, and tumor purging is not routinely performed. Arguments against purging include its cost and labor intensiveness. Moreover, for lymphoma and solid tumors, patients usually relapse at sites of prior bulky disease, suggesting that residual tumor within the recipient, not tumor in the stem cell product, is the primary contributor to relapse. Arguments in favor of purging include gene marking studies that show that marrow involvement can contribute to relapse.

ALLOGENEIC TRANSPLANTATION

Allogeneic transplantation uses stem cells from either a family member or an unrelated donor. Sources include bone marrow, peripheral blood, or umbilical cord blood.

- Typically fully matched donors are preferred, but various degrees of incompatibility can be tolerated with appropriate attention to prevention of rejection and graft-versus-host disease.

■ Haploidentical transplantation (from family members matched at one HLA haplotype, that is, potentially as few as 6/12 loci) is considered investigational.

High-Intensity Conditioning (Myeloablative) Transplantation

Allogeneic transplantation can control malignant disease by two distinct mechanisms. Like autologous transplantation, there is a dose-intensity component from the profound cytotoxicity of the conditioning regimen. In addition, the transplanted immune system can recognize mismatched minor histocompatibility antigens or tumor antigens expressed on tumor cells. The resultant anticancer effect is called the *graft-versus-malignancy effect* (this is commonly referred to as graft-versus-leukemia or graft-versus-lymphoma [GVL]). Thus, a myeloablative transplant is a two-pronged attack on the underlying disease and has a lower relapse rate than autologous transplantation. Unfortunately, the dose intensity of the conditioning may be prohibitively toxic for older patients or patients with comorbid disease, and early transplant-related mortality can be substantial. Moreover, dose intensity may predispose to more severe early GVHD.

Reduced-Intensity Conditioning Transplantation (Nonmyeloablative Transplantation)

The recognition of the contribution of GVL activity to disease eradication led to the development of reduced-intensity conditioning stem cell transplantation. Reduced-intensity transplantation is used for older patients or patients who are not eligible for myeloablative regimens (usually by virtue of age, comorbidities, or receipt of a prior autologous transplantation). These transplants are designed not to have direct antitumor activity, but rather to provide sufficient host immunosuppression to permit engraftment of donor hematopoietic and lymphoid effector cells. These effector cells can mediate a GVL effect responsible for tumor control. This type of transplantation is most appropriate either for diseases in remission (e.g., acute myeloid leukemia (AML) in complete remission) or for diseases that tend to be more indolent (e.g., chronic lymphoblastic leukemia (CLL), follicular lymphoma, myelofibrosis). More aggressive diseases generally require ablative transplantation unless they are performed when the disease is in complete remission.

PROS AND CONS OF EACH DONOR SOURCE

	Autologous	*Allogeneic*
Advantages	1. No HLA matching requirement	1. Stem cells have not been exposed to chemotherapy
	2. No GVHD	2. Stem cells product is free of tumor
	3. No need for immune suppression	3. Graft-versus-tumor activity
Disadvantages	1. Possibility of stem cell damage from prior therapy leading to delay in engraftment or MDS	1. Donor availability uncertain
	2. Possibility of contamination with tumor	2. GVHD
	3. No graft-versus-tumor effect	3. Higher risk of complications
	Lower risk of complications Higher risk of relapse	Higher risk of complications Lower risk of relapse

3. HLA MATCHING IN ALLOGENEIC TRANSPLANTATION

Understanding the human leukocyte antigen (HLA) system is critical for properly applying allogeneic stem cell transplantation. HLA loci are found on chromosome 6, and are generally inherited as complete haplotypes. Thus, any two siblings have a 25% chance of sharing two common parental haplotypes. However, crossovers can occasionally occur during chromosomal replication.

- Class I antigens – HLA-A, -B, and -C
  - HLA-A and -B are expressed on all cells. They are involved with antigen presentation to cytotoxic CD8$^+$ T cells, while HLA-C is implicated in natural killer (NK) antigen recognition. In the past, HLA-A and -B have been the only Class I antigens routinely typed for transplantation, but recently it has been demonstrated that disparity at the HLA-C locus may be associated with higher rates of graft rejection and graft-versus-host disease (GVHD) following unrelated stem cell transplantation.
  - Serologic methods are still used to type class I antigens, but more precise molecular methods are available and have led to more precise HLA typing than were previously available through serologic typing alone. In related transplants, serology is often adequate. The one exception is homozygosity of one of the antigens. In this case, there may be allele-level differences that need to be sorted out with molecular typing. In unrelated transplants, allele-level typing is preferable.
  - Through the use of allele-level typing, disease-free survival for matched unrelated hematopoietic stem cell transplantation (HSCT) is beginning to approach that for HSCT from HLA-identical siblings. However, rates of GVHD and nonrelapse mortality are still higher for recipients of unrelated marrow.
- Class II antigens – HLA-DR, DQ, and DP
  - Class II antigens are recognized by CD4$^+$ T cells. They are principally expressed on B cells, macrophages, and dendritic cells, and in some other cells to a more limited degree.

- It is clear that serologic typing is inadequate for class II typing, and molecular typing is employed routinely.
- HLA-DQ and DP are less important in allogeneic HSCT than HLA-DR, although some studies suggest a role for both in the pathogenesis of GVHD.

MINOR HISTOCOMPATIBILITY ANTIGENS

In addition to major HLA compatibility, there are also minor histocompatibility antigens that presumably have a role in GVHD, since transplantation with stem cells fully matched at both class I and class II HLA loci can still result in GVHD or rejection. Examples include HY antigens present on male but not female cells, HA1, HA2, and others.

HLA STATISTICS

In the United States, approximately 30% of patients have an HLA identical sibling. A smaller portion, less than 5%, will match a parent or an offspring. The likelihood of finding at least one match among n siblings is $1 - (0.75)^n$.

Number of Siblings	Probability of HLA Match
1	0.25
2	0.44
3	0.58
4	0.68

- The incidence of GVHD and graft failure increases with increasing HLA disparity. Generally, an unrelated donor is sought if a 5/6 HLA-A, B, DR matched relative cannot be found. There is some debate about whether a 6/6 unrelated donor is preferable to a 5/6 HLA-matched relative, but most feel that these donors are equivalent, and it is often easier from a logistic viewpoint to arrange the stem cell donation from a related donor.
- In umbilical cord blood transplantation, the immaturity of the donor immune system allows a greater degree of HLA disparity (e.g., 4/6 matches), although even here better matches are associated with better outcomes.

HLA TYPING

Patients and their siblings should be typed first. It is sometimes useful to type the patient's parents at the outset as well, if they are available, since it helps assign haplotypes and resolve inconsistencies in the siblings' typing. In the absence of a fully matched sibling, and in addition to doing an unrelated donor search, it may be useful to occasionally type children. If the children are very young, typing the patient's spouse can be useful, since one may avoid venipuncture in a child if analysis of the parents indicates that the child cannot match. Avoid typing extended family members unless there is a reasonable possibility that they match. Sometimes typing can be obtained from buccal swabs, which are easier to obtain from potential donors in some undeveloped countries.

4. STEM CELL SOURCE

HEMATOPOIETIC PROGENITOR CELL PRODUCTS

Hematopoietic progenitor cell (HPC) products contain hematopoietic stem and lineage-committed progenitor cells capable of providing hematopoietic and immune reconstitution after myeloablative or reduced-intensity preparative regimens. There is no unanimity on the terminology.

- Since stem cells are difficult to specifically identify, some authors prefer the term hematopoietic cell transplantation (HCT).
- Others call the procedure hematopoietic stem cell transplantation (HSCT) to acknowledge that most transplantations are not successful unless stem cells are transplanted.
- The Foundation For The Accreditation of Cellular Therapy (FACT) focuses on progenitors. Cellular therapy products can be broadly categorized as being minimally manipulated products and more than minimally manipulated products.

Hematopoietic Progenitor Cell Function

Hematopoietic progenitor cells (HPCs) administered intravenously migrate to the marrow, where they adhere, expand, self-renew (stem cells only), and differentiate. The differentiated cells are released into the blood, restoring blood counts and immunity. The time from administration of HPCs to recovery of adequate or normal blood counts is variable (see section on Engraftment).

Indications

Allogeneic HPC products are intended to provide hematopoietic reconstitution after myeloablative or reduced intensity preparative regimens for a wide range of disease states. For some patients the product is also intended to provide a graft-versus-tumor effect. Autologous HPCs are collected and stored for use as a "rescue" following myeloablative or severely myelotoxic therapy. The high-dose therapy is intended to treat the patient's underlying malignancy and autologous HPC products are administered to minimize morbidity and mortality due to the myelotoxic effects of the therapy.

Dosage and Administration

The minimum number of HPCs necessary for engraftment in a myeloablated recipient has not been established. Different products have widely different numbers of progenitors and stem cells. However, eligibility criteria for some protocols usually dictate a minimum number of cells to be collected and infused.

Several methods are used to measure the number of cells in an HPC collection. Simple cell count may be adequate for many marrow collections. Most centers use flow cytometric enumeration of $CD34^+$ cells for the majority of cellular products.

Storage

Hematopoietic progenitor cell (HPC) products are stored using various methods depending on the required duration of storage. Products used fresh can be refrigerated for at least 24 hours before infusion. If there is a >48-hour delay before infusion, most products are frozen to maintain viability. Most frozen products are stored in the vapor phase of liquid nitrogen ($\leq -50^{\circ}C$). Products may be stored for up to 10 years although no longevity limit has yet been determined. Long-term storage is generally done in the liquid phase of liquid nitrogen.

HEMATOPOIETIC PROGENITOR CELL SOURCES

Hematopoietic Progenitor Cell, Marrow

Hematopoietic progenitor cell, marrow (HPC-M) preparations contain HPCs obtained by multiple needle aspirations from the posterior iliac crest and occasionally from the anterior iliac crest or sternum of an autologous or allogeneic donor. The marrow is placed in a sterile container with an electrolyte solution and an appropriate anticoagulant. The cell suspension is passed through sterile filters to remove fat, bone particles, and cellular debris.

- The volume collected varies with the weight of the recipient, but generally ranges from 10 to 15 mL/kg of donor weight. The minimum nucleated cell dose is 2×10^8 nucleated cells/kg of recipient body weight.

- Marrow contains mature red cells, white cells, platelets, mast cells, fat cells, plasma cells, committed progenitors of all lineages, and HSC.
- These products are usually processed before infusion, but are sometimes infused in an unmodified state.
- The most common modifications of allogeneic HPC-M are to decrease the volume of ABO-incompatible red cells, remove ABO-incompatible plasma, isolate CD34$^+$ progenitor cells, and remove donor T lymphocytes.
- The most common modification of autologous HPC-M is to reduce the volume by removing plasma and red cells before cryopreservation.

Hematopoietic Progenitor Cell, Peripheral Blood

Hematopoietic progenitor cell, Apheresis (HPC-A) preparations contain HPCs collected from the peripheral blood by a leukapheresis procedure, usually after recombinant hematopoietic growth factor and/or chemotherapy administration.

- Mobilization regimens
  - *Granulocyte colony-stimulating factor (G-CSF).* 5 to 10 µg/kg SC per day (4 to 10 days, depending on the concomitant use of chemotherapy).
  - *Cytoxan plus G-CSF.* A single dose of 2,500 to 4,000 mg/m^2 IV with Mesna (used only in autologous transplantation) plus G-CSF 5 to 10 µg/kg SC per day for 4 to 10 days.
  - *Other.* Numerous chemotherapy regimens used to treat lymphoma can be used to mobilize stem cells. Stem cells are collected on recovery of neutrophils 10 to 14 days after chemotherapy.
  - *Mozobil (AMD3100, Plerixafor Hydrochloride).* Mozobil blocks CXCR4 (SDF-1α), facilitating release of hematopoietic progenitors and stem cells from the bone marrow and into the blood.
- Processing
  - An allogeneic HPC-A may be processed to decrease the volume of ABO-incompatible red cells, remove ABO-incompatible plasma, isolate CD34$^+$ progenitor cells, and remove donor T lymphocytes.
  - The most common modifications of autologous HPC-A are to reduce the volume by removing plasma before

cryopreservation, to isolate CD34$^+$ progenitor cells, and to wash the cells to remove DMSO after thawing.
■ The minimum CD34$^+$ cell dose is 2×10^6/kg.

Hematopoietic Progenitor Cell, Cord

Hematopoietic progenitor cell, cord (HPC-C) preparations contain HPCs obtained from the umbilical cord at the time of delivery. Cord blood products are used mainly for unrelated allogeneic stem cell transplantation. They may be used in family-member transplantation, particularly in children.

■ Initial processing may include removal of red cells and plasma. The HPC-C products are cryopreserved after collection and initial processing.
■ Cell dose is based per kilogram of recipient weight, which can be limiting. Target is 1.7 to 3.5×10^7 total nucleated cells/kg.
■ In adults, single cord blood unit transplantation is associated with very delayed engraftment, unless the recipient is small (below 40 kg). Combining two products seems to provide more rapid engraftment, albeit at the expense of higher rates of acute graft-versus-host disease (GVHD).

MINIMALLY MANIPULATED CELLULAR THERAPY PRODUCTS

Administration

The product should be administered or cryopreserved immediately after processing (within 48 hours of collection). It is filtered using a 170- to 260-micron filter. The infusion should be started slowly to observe for reactions and completed as quickly as tolerated. However, the administration time will be determined by the total volume to be infused and whether the cells are fresh or previously frozen.

PLASMA-REDUCED PRODUCTS

Description

These products contain the cellular elements of the HPCs that remain after the bulk of the plasma is removed by centrifugation.

Plasma depletion is performed only for minor ABO-incompatible products ($O \Rightarrow A$; $O \Rightarrow B$; $O \Rightarrow AB$; $B \Leftrightarrow A$; $B \Rightarrow AB$; $A \Rightarrow AB$) with plasma volume greater than 150 mL.

Indications

Plasma-reduced HPC graft is indicated

- when the donor has an antibody to one or more recipient red cell antigens, such as in minor ABO-incompatible situations;
- as a means of volume reduction for recipients who are small, fluid-sensitive, or have preexisting fluid overload, cardiac or renal compromise;
- autologous HPCs collected by apheresis are plasma-reduced to decrease volume before cryopreservation.

RED CELL–REDUCED PRODUCTS

Description

These are the HPCs remaining after the mature red cells have been depleted by sedimentation, centrifugation, or lysis. Red blood cell depletion is performed only for major ABO-incompatible products ($A \Rightarrow O$; $B \Rightarrow O$; $AB \Rightarrow O$; $A \Leftrightarrow B$) or for patients with other clinically significant antibodies, and when the total red blood cell (RBC) content is greater than 30 mL.

Indications

- The recipient may have a high-titer antibody to one or more antigens on the donor red cells (usually major ABO incompatibility).
- Red cell depletion is also used to reduce the concentration of an autologous HPC product before cryopreservation.

BUFFY COAT ENRICHED PRODUCTS

Description

The buffy coat is the portion of an HPC product containing the nucleated cells after the bulk of the plasma and mature red cells have been removed by sedimentation or centrifugation techniques.

Indications

This procedure is indicated when a concentrated HPC product is required for further manipulation such as purging and/or cryo-preservation. It may also be used when greater volume reduction is desired than can be obtained with plasma reduction alone.

CRYOPRESERVED PRODUCTS

Description

Cryopreserved products are HPCs that have been frozen using cryoprotectant solutions. The most commonly used cyryprotectant is 10% DMSO and a protein additive such as human serum albumin.

Indications

Cryopreservation of cells is indicated when the product is to be stored for more than 48 hours before administration.

Administration

- The product should be administered immediately after thawing and/or processing. Cell death occurs rapidly after the product is thawed. A 2-hour expiration from time of thaw on most routine cryopreserved HPC products is reasonable but may be center dependent.
- All products should be filtered at the bedside using a 170- to 260-micron filter.
- The infusion should be started slowly to observe for reactions and completed as quickly as tolerated. However, the administration time will be determined by the total volume to be infused.
- If the thawed products have not been washed to remove DMSO, care should be taken not to exceed 1mL of DMSO per kilogram of recipient weight per day administration (e.g., 100 mL of 10% solution contains 10 mL of DMSO).

CD34-ENRICHED PRODUCTS

Description

CD34-enriched products contain the cellular elements of HPCs that have been enriched by CD34 selection.

Indications

A CD34-enriched HPC product may be indicated

- when circulating tumor cells are present in the peripheral blood and/or marrow and, therefore, will likely be present in the HPC product;
- as a means to reduce the number of T lymphocytes contained in the allogeneic HPC product.

5. PRETRANSPLANT EVALUATION AND COUNSELING OF PATIENT AND DONOR

PRETRANSPLANT COUNSELING

Both patient and donor are completely evaluated before stem cell transplantation. The evaluation should comply within guidelines established by the Food and Drug Administration (FDA), Foundation for the Accreditation of Cellular Therapy (FACT), and other regulations and should be available in written form specific to your institution. Both patient and donor evaluations include a thorough history and physical examination and a series of studies to confirm medical eligibility.

Treatment recommendations should be discussed thoroughly with the patient, donor, and family. The marrow graft procedure as well as alternative forms of therapy, as far as they exist, should be presented as objectively as possible. The risks and hazards of stem cell mobilization and the donation procedure and any other procedures associated with the donation must be explained to the donor as well as to the patient or, in the case of minors, to the donor or patient's responsible family member. Plans for protection of fertility are also discussed at this time. Reading material, videotapes, and other education aides are helpful and should be available. In addition, a discussion of patient wishes regarding aggressive supportive measures (i.e., cardiopulmonary resuscitation, mechanical ventilation, other artificial means of life support), and establishment of a living will or other advanced directives should be included at this time. It is important to point out specifically that some aspects of hematopoietic stem cell transplantation (HSCT) are still considered experimental. We strongly recommend that patients undergo a psychosocial evaluation and that financial aspects of the transplant are discussed with the patient and his/her family before transplantation.

PATIENT PRETRANSPLANT EVALUATION

It is appropriate that a consultation with a transplant physician and insurance approval are obtained before an unrelated donor search is initiated. Keep in mind that insurance companies may pay for the transplantation but not for search costs or critical prescription drugs needed for prolonged periods of time. This can lead to considerable stress for both the patient and clinical team and a plan should be put in place early in the evaluation.

Restaging, eligibility, and pre-HSCT workup must be completed within a specific time based on individual institution's registration policy (protocols may be specific). Exceptions should require specific exemption by the HSCT program medical director and must be documented. FACT guidelines require that infectious disease marker testing be completed within 30 days before donation for allogeneic and autologous marrow and peripheral blood stem cell transplant (PBSC) donors and 7 days before donation for allogeneic lymphocyte donors. FACT also requires that pregnancy testing be performed within 7 days before the initiation of recipient's conditioning regimen or of donor starting mobilization regimen.

Recommended Patient Workup

1. Complete physical examination including neurological assessment and performance status.
2. Complete history, including cultures: recreational drug use, alcohol, positive blood culture with current central venous lines (CVL), transfusion, pregnancies, abortions, recent travel, vaccinations. Social history is particularly important to establish reliability of caretakers and home environment.
3. Blood workup: CBC, differential blood count, complete panel, lipid profile, LDH, ferritin, TSH, PT/PTT, blood type and screen, ß-HCG should be obtained for patients <55 years of age and potentially fertile; human leukocyte antigen (HLA) typing, for allogeneic transplant, Creatinine clearance (CrCl) is helpful.
4. Infection disease testing (serologies): cytomegalovirus (CMV), Hep A, Hep BsAg, HBc antibody, Hep B sAb, HCV antibody, HIV I and II, HIV ag (NAT testing preferred), HTLV-1 and 2 antibody, RPR, HSV 1&2, Epstein-Barr virus (EBV), varicella zoster virus (VZV), toxoplasmosis.
5. Additional testing: GFR scan if known renal insufficiency or unable to collect CrCl, RVG or ECHO w/EF, EKG, CXR, PFTs w/DLCO. Consider sinus CT for patients with history of sinusitis (helpful to specify coronal views), nasal passage aspirate/washing for respiratory virus if symptoms present,

stool for *Clostridium difficile* if there is a positive history or symptoms.

6. Purified protein derivative (PPD) screening: All HSCT candidates should have a PPD placed as early as possible before transplant; 5 mm of induration is considered positive in an immunocompromised patient. A 10 mm induration is considered positive independent of BCG vaccination status, unless they are foreign-born from a country with very low incidence of TB. Controls such as mumps or candida are on no value and likely to lead to misinterpretations and should not be used.

- All HSCT candidates should have a chest radiograph. Evidence of prior TB such as a Ghon complex without a positive PPD should be handled identically as in patients with positive PPD who have never received therapy, unless there is an alternative explanation for their findings.
- Prevention of clinical TB is extremely important in highly immunocompromised HSCT recipients who have been exposed to someone with active pulmonary TB regardless of the PPD status and in highly immunocompromised HSCT recipients who have a positive PPD but who were not previously treated and who have no evidence of active TB.

Prevention options:

INH 300 mg/day orally × 9 months (270 doses) and pyridoxine 25 to 50 mg orally daily.

Twice weekly schedule of INH and pyridoxine. INH 900 mg orally twice per week and pyridoxine 50 to 100 mg orally twice per week.

- Patients who cannot receive or tolerate the aforementioned regimen should be referred to an infectious disease specialist for evaluation and consideration of alternative regimens.
- Ideally, transplantation should not be scheduled until at least 2 weeks after completion of therapy. For patients in whom HSCT should not be delayed because of the underlying disease process and have no evidence of active TB, treatment can be initiated after discharge from the hospital or at day + 28 at the latest. If INH described earlier cannot be administered, infectious disease consultation should be obtained for advice on an alternative regimen.

7. Restaging studies: bone marrow aspirate, $+/-$ cytogenetics, LP, CT/MRI, gallium or PET scan, HLA typing as appropriate.

8. Recommended patient pretransplant consults:

    a   Radiation therapy consult for total body irradiation (TBI) and lung block films. May also need cranial irradiation or total lymphocyte irradiation (TLI)

    b   Dental evaluation and prophylaxis (within 6 months before admission)

    c   Fertility: sperm banking or oocyte or embryo freezing

    d   Social service

    e   Psychiatry (as needed)

    f   Dietary consult as needed.

9. Suggested patient education and informed consent:

    a   Information session with a transplant program physician, nurse, NP (nurse practitioner) or PA (physician assistant) who will provide the patient with reading material, videotapes, educational tools, and information regarding the need for central venous catheter placement including home care, if necessary, associated risks and discomfort.

    b   Financial aspects of the transplant.

    c   Consent appointment with transplant attending physician.

In all cases, patients should be informed of their infectious disease markers. Such notification should always be conducted within standard confidentiality guidelines. Patients with evidence of infection should be referred to the appropriate primary care physician or specialist before transplantation.

DONOR ELIGIBILITY AND MEDICAL SUITABILITY

Donors must be evaluated to ensure that the stem cell product is safe for HSCT recipients, that the process of donation will not cause harm to the donor, and that they understand completely what they are being asked to do.

Donor evaluations should comply with both FDA regulations 21, Part 1271 and FACT-JACIE International Standards. The National Marrow Donor Program (NMDP) provides action forms that can be used as a tool to help determine donor eligibility. The following is a general overview of determining donor eligibility and is not to be considered comprehensive. Refer to your institute's standard operating procedures as well as FDA, State, FACT, AABB, and NMDP guidelines.

Recommended Donor Work-Up

1. Complete physical examination, including evaluation for safety risks of the collection procedure in the possible need for central venous access and/or mobilization therapy for collection of blood cells and anesthesia for the collection of marrow.

2. Complete history and physical examination including history of the following: recreational drug use, alcohol, hypertension, cigarette smoking, blood transfusion, pregnancies, abortions, recent travel, vaccinations, and malignant disease. To identify persons at risk for transmission of communication disease (as defined by the FDA), inherited conditions, and/or hematological or immunological disease, the donor must also complete an Allogeneic Donor Health History Questionnaire (HHQ) form per the FDA. Completion of this form along with a series of studies can be used to determine medical eligibility and suitability.

3. Blood workup: CBC, differential counts, complete panel, LDH, PT/PTT, blood type, and screen (at blood bank), HLA testing, and β-hCG assessment should be obtained for female donors of childbearing potential.

4. Infectious disease testing (serologies): labs must be drawn within 30 days before stem cell or marrow collection. Labs includeCMV Ab IgG, EBV, and an infectious disease marker (IDM) panel (HIV-1 and -2 antibody, HIV antigen NAT, HTLV-1 and -2 antibody, WNV NAT, HbsAg, HBcAb, HCV NAT, RPR, CMV and type and screen). IDM panel must be tested according to FDA standards.

5. Additional recommended testing if clinically indicated, urinalysis, chest X-ray, and/or EKG. EKG required for marrow donors males >40 years, females >50 years. PPD for all donors with appropriate risk factors (valid for 6 months before donation).

6. Repeat donors: repeat donors should be evaluated according to FDA and institutional standards.

7. Donor education and appointments:

   ▪ Donor education recommendations:
   – During medical examination all donors should be informed not to ingest potential bone marrow

suppressive agents such as ETOH or antiplatelet drugs such as asprin for at least 2 weeks before donation. No nonsteroidal anti-inflammatory medications for 24 hours before donation.
- Provide reading material.
- Provide an impartial donor advocate available upon request.

- ▦ Donor appointment recommendations:
  - Information session scheduled
  - Consult and informed consent session with HSCT trained clinician
  - Social worker or psychosocialconsult before donation if necessary
  - PBSC donors only – evaluation of peripheral access by an apheresis nurse
  - PBSC donors only – mobilization therapy administration information appointment with qualified donor center staff nurse
  - Marrow donors only – anesthesia consult
  - Marrow donors only – phlebotomy $\times$ 1 or 2 for an autologous use of donor blood

8. Donor consent: a consult and informed consent session should be scheduled with an HSCT trained clinician before the high-dose therapy of the patient is initiated.

- ▦ All forms must be signed before the high-dose therapy of the patient is initiated.
- ▦ During the informed consent visit with the donor, or in case of minors, the donor and donor's responsible family member, the clinician should
  - describe the differences between cells derived from HPC sources (marrow vs. PB or lymphocytes if DLI donor);
  - explain the risks, benefits, and alternatives associated with donation of each form of HPC product;
  - review and explain individualized risks to the donor, if applicable, as indicated by the donor's full health history and physical evaluation;
  - indicate whether the HPC product is to be frozen for any reason;
  - review the institute or hospital's policy for storage and disposition of unused frozen products;

- – answer donor's questions;
- – obtain consent and authorization in advance to release the donor's health information relevant to the safe conduct of the transplant, to the transplant physician and patient;
- – explain that the donor has the right to refuse to donate and to review the results of tests performed to determine donor's eligibility status;
- – inform the donor of alternatives to donation;
- – plan for appropriate postdonation care;
  - ▣ FACT and FDA documentation and consent requirements should be followed.
9. Review of donor data and completion of forms should be followed per FDA and FACT standards.
   - ▣ An interim health assessment of donor suitability is obtained and documented immediately before each collection procedure.
10. Repeat testing and documentation requirements for donors with workups that are outdated; should follow FDA and FACT guidelines.

6. CONDITIONING REGIMENS

Conditioning regimens are designed to destroy tumor cells resistant to conventional doses of chemotherapy without causing fatal nonhematologic organ toxicity. In patients undergoing allogeneic stem cell transplantation, conditioning regimens must be sufficiently immunosuppressive to prevent the recipient from mounting an immune response capable of rejecting the graft. Graft rejection is uncommon, but this complication is associated with a dire outcome and the risk increases with the degree of mismatch.

There are few randomized trials comparing different ablative regimens; in general, increased intensity of the conditioning regimen may decrease relapse rates but usually (though not always) at the expense of increased nonrelapse morbidity and mortality. The following represent some of the more common regimens used today, although different combinations and doses may be used at different centers. It is essential to check the specific protocol that applies to the patient for drugs, doses, frequency, and other specifics of treatments. Biologic agents such as Campath or antithymocyte globulin (ATG) may be added to enhance immunosuppression. See Appendix for ideal body weight (IBW) and adjusted ideal body weight (AIBW) for obese patients.

Regimen	Comment
CBV – cyclophosphamide, BCNU, etoposide	Typically used in autologous transplantation for lymphoproliferative disorders
Bu/Cy – busulfan, cyclophosphamide	Common regimen used in allogeneic SCT. Frequently used in autologous SCT for AML. Busulfan can be given IV or orally. Pharmacokinetic monitoring is used to limit toxicity
Cy/TBI – cyclophosphamide, total body irradiation	Most commonly used in allogeneic SCT. Probably more effective for ALL than Bu/Cy
BEAM – BCNU, etoposide, Ara-c, melphalan	Typically used in autologous transplantation for lymphoproliferative disorders
Melphalan	Used exclusively in myeloma

(*continued*)

Regimen	Comment
Flu/Bu – fludarabine, busulfan	Typically used for allogeneic SCT. It can be used in high-dose or reduced-intensity regimens
Flu/Mel – fludarabine, melphalan	Typically used for allogeneic SCT. It can be used in high-dose or reduced-intensity regimens
Fludarabine, low-dose TBI	Typically used for reduced-intensity allogeneic SCT

AGENTS

Antithymocyte Globulin

Mechanism of Action
Immune suppressant – destroys thymus-dependent human T cells and other immune cells (natural killer [NK] cells, dendritic cells) responsible for cellular-mediated immunity.

Dose
- Thymoglobulin (Genzyme) 1.5 mg/kg daily × 4 days.
- ATGAM (Upjohn) 30 to 40 mg/kg daily × 4 to 5 days.

There is no single accepted dose. These doses are sugges-tions. It is of note that the dose of ATG here differs from the dose used as therapy for steroid-refractory graft-versus-host disease (GVHD).

Indication
- Aplastic anemia.
- Some ablative and nonablative conditioning regimens for malignancies include ATG to both deplete residual host T cells and because residual ATG will reduce the effective dose of infused T cells with the graft.[1]

Administration
At a slow rate at first to monitor for reactions and then the rate may be increased. Use benadryl and/or corticosteroids as premedication.

Toxicity
IMMEDIATE
These include rare fatal allergic reactions. Fevers, chills, hypotension, and third-spacing including pulmonary edema and prerenal azotemia are common. Reversible hepatic dysfunction.

DELAYED
Skin rash and joint pains (serum sickness) can occur.

BCNU (Carmustine)

Mechanism of Action
Cell phase nonspecific. Causes DNA cross-links and strand breaks. It carbamoylates cellular proteins and inhibits DNA repair.

Metabolism
Plasma half-life is 1 hour. Approximately 70% of the IV dose is excreted in urine within 96 hours of administration. Significant concentrations remain in the cerebrospinal fluid (CSF) for 9 hours because of lipid solubility.

Dose
112.5 mg/m^2/day for 4 days as part of CBV regimen mentioned earlier.

Administration
IV bolus given over 30 minutes.

Side Effects
IMMEDIATE
■   Nausea, vomiting, reversible hepatic dysfunction, infusion reaction (hypotension, especially with high dose dissolved in 10% ethanol).

DELAYED/CUMULATIVE
■   Nephrotoxcity: Cumulative doses (>1,000 mg/m^2)
■   Pulmonary toxicity: Dose-related if cumulative dose >600 mg/m^2. Other risk factors include abnormal pulmonary function tests before transplant (baseline forced vital capacity (FVC) <70% of predicted; carbon monoxide diffusion capacity (DLCO) <70% of predicted) or if a patient is

receiving concurrent cyclophosphamide or thoracic radiation. Symptoms include cough, dyspnea, tachypnea, and restrictive-type ventilatory defect. Chest X-ray may show interstitial infiltrates. Acute pulmonary toxicity (day 10 to 30 after HSCT) is responsive to steroids.

Busulfan

Mechanism of Action
It is an alkylating agent. Forms carbonium ions through the release of a methane sulfonate group, resulting in the alkylation of DNA. Acts primarily on the granulocyte precursors in the bone marrow and is cell cycle, phase nonspecific.

Metabolism
This drug is 32% protein bound. Metabolized by the liver and excreted in the urine (30%). Metabolites may be long-lived. When administered IV, equal concentrations appear in the plasma and CSF.

Dose
Previously it was only administered orally. However, IV busulfan (Busulfex) has replaced oral therapy in many centers. It is critical to perform pharmacokinetic monitoring when using oral dosing.

ABLATIVE REGIMEN
Busulfex 0.8 mg/kg (IBW or actual weight, whichever is lower) IV every 6 hours over 3 hours for 4 days (total of 16 doses). Drug clearance is best predicted when busulfan dose is based on adjusted ideal body weight. See Appendix for IBW and AIBW calculations. Seizure prophylaxis with levetiracetam is recommended because there are no drug interactions with busulfan. No loading dose is given and levels are not monitored.

NONMYELOABLATIVE REGIMEN
Busulfex 0.8 mg/kg IV QD or BID

Administration
Infuse dose over 2 to 3 hours via infusion pump and through a central line.

Toxicity

IMMEDIATE

- ■ Neurotoxicity: Drug crosses the blood–brain barrier and lowers seizure threshold. Prophylaxis with levetiracetam as mentioned earlier. Note that phenytoin administration can affect cyclosporine, tacrolimus, and rapamycin levels (decreasing levels by inducing P450 metabolism).
- ■ Gastrointestinal: Nausea, vomiting, diarrhea, stomatitis, anorexia. Hepatitis and veno-occlusive disease (VOD) are more common with high-dose regimens.
- ■ Skin: Hyperpigmentation, rash, alopecia. Hair loss may be permanent.

DELAYED

- ■ Pulmonary: Pulmonary fibrosis can occur 4 months to 10 years post therapy. Average onset is 4 years post therapy.
- ■ Sexual Dysfunction: Premenopausal female patients often experience ovarian suppression and amenorrhea with menopausal symptoms. Men experience sterility, azoospermia, and testicular atrophy. The drug is a potential teratogen.

Cyclophosphamide (Cytoxan/Cy/Ctx)

Mechanism of Action
Alkylating agent. Causes cross-linking of DNA strands and prevents DNA synthesis and cell division. Cell cycle phase nonspecific.

Metabolism
The drug is inactive until microsomes in the liver and serum enzymes (phosphamidases) convert to active form. Both the inactive form and its metabolites are excreted by the kidneys. Half-life is 6 to 12 hours. Approximately 25% of the drug is excreted after 8 hours. Plasma half-life is increased in patients with renal failure.

Dose
The dose ranges from 1.8 to 6 g/m². 1800 mg/m² IV daily for 2 days or 60 mg/kg/day for 2 days or 1500 mg/m² for 2 to 4 days (Bu/Cy aplastic anemia regimen and CBV).

Administration
Prepare in 500 cc normal saline. High doses should be given over 60 minutes. Prehydrate with 1000 cc D5NS plus 20 mEq of

potassium at 500 cc/hr for 2 hours predose and then D51/2NS at 200 cc/hr. Maintain urine output of 200 cc/hr (using furosemide if necessary). Alternatively, Mesna can be used to prevent hemorrhagic cystitis with high doses proceeding, during and for 24 hours following CTX administration.

Drug Interactions

Increased myelosuppression when given with thiazide diuretics; decreases digoxin absorption; can potentiate trastuzumab, and doxorubicin-induced cardiomyopathy. CYP2B6 and 3A4 inducers (phenytoin, phenobarbital, rifampin, etc.) increase acrolein (cyclophosphamide metabolite) levels: CYP2B6 and 3A4 inhibitors (sertraline, desipramine, azole antifungals, etc.) decrease acrolein levels.

Toxicity

IMMEDIATE

- Histamine reaction may occur with rapid administration. Symptoms may include burning nose, facial pain, lip tingling. The reaction responds rapidly to diphenhydramine or benztropine
- Cardiovascular toxicity: Cardiomyopathy, hemorrhagic cardiac necrosis, and coronary artery vasculitis may occur with high doses. Hemorrhagic myopericarditis may cause cardiac tamponade. Signs and symptoms include CHF, tamponade, or arrhythmia.
- Genitourinary toxicity: Hemorrhagic cystitis can occur if metabolites of the drug are allowed to accumulate. This is preventable with sufficient hydration or administration of Mesna with high doses. Hydration minimizes the contact of mucosa with acrolein. Mesna binds to the active metabolite, preventing injury to the bladder mucosa. Mesna is effective only during CTX metabolism/excretion and not if hemorrhagic cystitis is a later sequela of CTX. Cystitis presents as dysuria, usually with either microscopic or gross hematuria. Long-term drug exposure may lead to bladder fibrosis. For additional information on cystitis see Chapter 23, cystitis.
- Endocrine toxicity: SIADH with water retention from direct action on renal tubules, which can lead to hyponatremia and seizures. Diagnosis is based on the following:
  - Euvolemic or mildly hypervolemic, hypoosmolality, inappropriately increased urine osm, urine sodium >40 mg/L, low BUN, and UA.

- – Differential diagnosis of SIADH: Medications (cyclophosphamide, antidepressants, antipsychotics, thiazides), pulmonary process, intracranial process, endocrinopathies (adrenal insufficiency and hypothyroid), surgery, tumors, psychogenic polydipsia other (pain, nausea, postop states).
  - – Treatment: Free water restriction and treat underlying cause if possible.
- ■ Gastrointestinal toxicity: Nausea and vomiting. Typically begins 2 to 4 hours after dose and peaks at 12 hours. Anorexia is common. Stomatitis is usually mild. Hepatotoxicity is rare.
- ■ Skin toxicity: Hair loss occurs in all patients. Alopecia in 30% to 50%. Hyperpigmentation and transverse ridging of nails (banding) can occur.
- ■ Pulmonary toxicity: Rare, but may occur with very high doses or continuous low-dose therapy. Onset is insidious. Appears as interstitial pneumonitis, which may progress to fibrosis. Steroids may be of benefit.

Etoposide (VP-16)

Mechanism of Action
Topoisomerase II inhibitor. It inhibits DNA synthesis in S and G2 phase of the cell cycleso that cells are unable to enter mitosis, and it causes single-strand breaks in DNA.

Metabolism
Rapidly excreted in urine and to a lesser extent in bile. Approximately 30% of drug is excreted unchanged. The majority binds to albumin and becomes tissue bound.

Administration
Infuse over 1 to 4 hours to minutes to minimize risk of acute hypersensitivity.

Dose
75 to 2400 mg/m^2 IV or 10 to 60 mg/kg. Dose will vary per protocol or treatment plan.

Special Considerations
Reduce dose by 50% if bilirubin >1.5 mg/dL and 75% if bilirubin >3.0 mg/dL. Reduce drug by 25% if creatinine clearance 10 to 50 mL/min.

Toxicity

IMMEDIATE

■ Acute hypersensitivity including anaphylaxis or anaphylactoid reactions. Decrease rate and use additional premedications such as benadryl.

■ Gastrointestinal toxicity: Nausea and vomiting occur shortly after infusion. Hepatitis, stomatitis, and metabolic acidosis may occur at high doses.

■ Skin toxicity: Rash, especially if patient has had prior radiation therapy (radiation recall phenomenon). Rash may be maculopapular, nodular, or bullous. Plantar and palmar burning may occur.

■ Cardiovascular toxicity: Myocardial infarction has been very rarely reported in patients who have had prior mediastinal XRT and patients receiving etoposide-containing regimens. Arrhythmias are uncommon. Patients with coronary artery disease may be at greater risk.

Fludarabine Phosphate

Mechanism of Action

Inhibits DNA synthesis, probably by inhibiting DNA-polymerase-α, ribonucleotide reductase.

Metabolism

Purine analogue; antimetabolite which is metabolized to 2-fluoroara-adenosine when given IV. Drug half-life is about 10 hours. Route of elimination is through the kidneys. Approximately 20% to 25% is excreted unchanged in the urine.

Administration

IV bolus over 30 minutes. May vary by protocol.

Dose

25 to 30 mg/m^2 IV daily $\times$ 4 to 5 days.

Toxicity

This drug is generally very well tolerated.

■ Immediate toxicity: Gastrointestinal: Nausea, vomiting, and diarrhea.

Melphalan

Mechanism of Action
Alkylating agent. Prevents cell replication by causing breaks and cross-linkages in DNA strands causing miscoding and breakage. Cell-cycle phase nonspecific.

Metabolism
Half-life approximately 2 hours. Excreted in feces over 6 days and urine within 24 hours.

Administration
Infuse over 15 to 30 minutes, as specified by protocol.

Dose
Ranges from 50 to 200 mg/m²/day. Dose will vary per protocol or treatment plan.

Toxicity
- Gastrointestinal toxicity: Nausea, vomiting, stomatitis.
- Skin toxicity: Rashes.
- Pulmonary toxicity: Pulmonary toxicity following interstitial pneumonitis and fibrosis. In most cases, the effects have been reversible.

Total Body Irradiation

Dose
Will vary per protocol and treatment plan. A common range is 175 to 200 cGy BID for 4 days (1200 to 1400 cGy total). If indicated, cranial boost pretransplant may be administered the week before admission, generally for patients with acute lymphoblastic leukemia or patients with prior central nervous system (CNS) involvement.

Side Effects
IMMEDIATE
- Fatigue, nausea, vomiting, rash (diffuse mild erythema)
- Parotitis (elevated amylase, normal lipase)
- Sterility

- Pulmonary: Acute pneumonitis (diffuse alveolar hemorrhage, DAH)

DELAYED
- Growth failure, thyroid dysfunction, gonadal failure
- Cataracts
- Renal dysfunction

PREVENTION OF COMPLICATIONS OF CONDITIONING THERAPY

There are a few generally accepted methods of preventing conditioning-related complications. Clearly, attention to dosing and schedule are critical. For the most part, rather than "side effects," the conditioning regimen toxicity can be considered the undesirable effects of the agents on normal organs.

- Skin toxicity: Patients receiving TBI should not use skin moisturizers, lotions, creams, deodorants, or any topical medications, since the emoliants and lubricants tend to exacerabate skin injury.
- Menstrual bleeding: Menstruating women may receive lupron at least one month before conditioning therapy begins. Since most conditioning regimens cause amenorrhea, the dose may not need to be repeated. Although oral estrogens and progestins may be used to treat vaginal bleeding, the estrogens may cause liver function abnormalities. Moreover, erratic use of these agents can result in a "confused uterus," which may exacerbate the problem. Our recommendation is that mild to moderate vaginal bleeding does not require intervention. More severe bleeding may respond to lo-ovral 2 to 4 tablets daily until bleeding stops then 1 tablet daily. Megace 40 mg po QID is also an option and may be less nauseating and less hepatotoxic than estrogen tablets. Intramuscular injections during HSCT are to be avoided.
- Urinary bleeding: Different approaches may be used but most commonly hydration as described earlier or the use of Mesna to prevent cyclophosphamide cardiotoxicity.
- CNS: High-dose busulfan may be associated with seizures and levoracetam (Keppra) may be useful as prophylaxis.

MUCOSITIS

Kepivance may be used with highly mucotoxic regimens. The recommended dosage of Kepivance is 60 µg/kg/day, administered as an IV bolus injection for 3 consecutive days before and 3 consecutive days after myelotoxic therapy for a total of 6 doses. The most common serious adverse reaction attributed to Kepivance is rash, which occurs in less than 5% of cases. Oral dysesthesia, tongue discoloration, tongue thickening, alteration of taste may occur within a week of starting.

REFERENCE

1. Armand P, Antin JH. Allogeneic stem cell transplantation for aplastic anemia. *Biol Blood Marrow Transplant.* 2007 May;13(5):505–516.

7. STEM CELL INFUSION

AUTOLOGOUS

Stem cells are routinely cryopreserved with dimethyl sulfoxide (DMSO). These products are red blood cell (RBC) depleted before cryopreservation and thawed at 37°C water bath before infusion. They should be infused through standard 170-micron red blood cell filters.

GENERAL REACTIONS AND RESPONSE TO INFUSION TOXICITY

The infusion of hematopoietic stem cells may be associated with toxicities that are either specific to hematopoietic products or general to all blood product infusions. The following text provides a minimal guideline to the workup and management of infusional toxicities. Each anticipated toxicity is defined and a plan of action is outlined.

Bleeding

- Unprocessed marrow contains approximately 20,000 units of heparin, which is infused over 1 to 4 hours. This will result in anticoagulation to a degree sufficient to result in clinical bleeding. Patients at risk are those with a history of recent surgery (e.g., recent line placement or revision), hemorrhagic cystitis, severe thrombocytopenia. However, bleeding can occur in any individual.
- For a patient with a known hemorrhagic risk, the marrow should be concentrated and washed to remove heparin. If the risk factor is known before a harvest takes place, acid citrate dextrose (ACD) can be used in place of heparin as a cryopreservative, if allowed by protocol.
- Infused heparin can be reversed with protamine. One mg of protamine will neutralize approximately 100 units of heparin. Maximum dose is 50 mg and the infusion rate should not exceed 5 mg/minute.

Fevers

- Fevers after infusion of stem cell and blood products can be due to bacterial contamination of the product. Often stem cells have a long travel period before infusion, giving skin contaminants an opportunity to grow. Severe fevers, hypotension, or evidence of sepsis needs to be treated aggressively until cultures are either negative or establish an organism.
- Fevers may be due to contaminated product, cytokines released during collection and processing, or infection coincidental to stem cell infusion.
- Low-grade fevers can be observed if there is no rigor, hypotension, or systemic symptoms suggestive of infection. The marrow infusion should be completed. The use of antibiotics and/or antipyretics should be up to the treating physician.
- High fevers (>100.5) should result in the collection of blood cultures and stem cell product culture. It is generally prudent to start broad-spectrum antibiotics until cultures are known to be negative and the patient has defervesced and is clinically stable.

Fluid Overload

- Fluid overload should be treated by slowing the infusion and treating with diuretics as clinically indicated.

DMSO Toxicity

- DMSO toxicity (nausea, vomiting, erythema, headache, pruritis, dizziness, bad-taste in mouth, changes in blood pressure, heart rate) can generally be treated by slowing the rate of infusion. Occasionally, hypotension will require the use of volume expansion. This is typically accomplished with a rapid saline infusion. If severe or not corrected in 20 minutes, consider dopamine. If symptoms are severe the product should have the DMSO removed.
- DMSO-preserved product has a distinctive odor (charitably described as "garlic"). It can persist in the patient's room for 48 to 72 hours.
- Mild intravascular hemolysis may occur due to remaining RBCs in marrow collection. Urine tests may be positive for

hemoglobin for 24 to 48 hours. This is commonly associated with a rise in serum lactate dehydrogenase (LDH). Maintain hydration and follow creatinine.

- Arrhythmias such as atrial fibrillation and bradycardia can occur. Hypotension, hypertension, and renal insufficiency can occur. Headache, nausea, vomiting are common. All patients should have cardiac monitoring during stem cell infusion. If arrhythmia is unresponsive to usual treatment measures, it is recommended to involve a cardiologist for management.

- It is recommended that the amount of DMSO be limited to 40 mL/day regardless of the patient's weight. If several products are stored, infusions can either be spread out over more than one day or the DMSO can be washed out.

Acute Hemolytic Transfusion Reaction

- A standard blood transfusion reaction investigation should be initiated.
- Hydrate the patient to ensure rapid urine flow. If necessary, augment with lasix or mannitol.
- If DIC is present treat with platelets, fresh frozen plasma (FFP), and transfusions as clinically indicated.

Patent Foramen Ovale

Approximately 10% of the population has a patent foramen ovale (PFO). This is generally not a problem. However, in some patients with increased right-sided pressures there may be R→L blood flow. Infusion of stem cell products, especially, if a filter is not used can result in cerebral emboli because of cell aggregates in the product. We recommend using a standard blood filter for all stem cell products that may have cellular or fibrin aggregates.

8. ABO COMPATIBILITY

Whenever possible, donors who are ABO compatible with the recipient should be selected. However, since human leukocyte antigen (HLA) and ABO types are unrelated, it is common to have HLA compatible donors who are ABO incompatible. This disparity often requires special attention. Transfusion problems may occur immediately or after a delay.

Soon after birth, antibodies form against bacterial polysaccharides that cross-react with ABO substance. Thus, type A people have anti-B antibodies without ever being exposed to type B blood. Similarly, type B people have anti-A antibodies and type O people have antibodies to both A and B, while type AB people have no antibodies. Immediate transfusion risk is due to this preformed antibody reacting with infused red blood cells (RBCs) during the stem cell product infusion. Delayed reactions reflect slow turnover of plasma cells or antibody weeks or months after the transplant, resulting in delayed erythroid recovery. When considering transfusion risks, both the red cell type and the associated antibodies must be considered. Donor recipient pairs are defined as follows:

MAJOR MISMATCH

As shown in the following table, if the recipient is type O and the donor is type A, B, or AB, there is a major ABO incompatibility. In this situation, there are preformed antibodies in the type O recipient against A and/or B substance on the donor's RBCs.

Transfusion of the unmodified stem cell product can result in an acute hemolytic transfusion reactions (AHTR). This type of reaction can manifest in multiple ways, pain at the IV sight, hypo/hypertension, fever, back or flank pain, gross hematuria.

After an otherwise successful transplant, some patients will have prolonged failure of erythropoiesis. If the recipient is a high-titer antibody producer (primarily anti-A), he or she may maintain high titers of antibody long after otherwise successful engraftment. This appears functionally to be a form of pure red cell aplasia since the antibody destroys red cells or red cell precursors in the marrow before they enter the circulation.

MINOR MISMATCH

In this setting the donor is type O and the recipient is A, B, or AB. Normally this does not result in any immediate problems since the type O red cells will not react with preformed antibody in the recipient. However, there are some data that the preformed antibody in the type O donor's plasma can cause problems[1] – including nonspecific organ injury (veno-occlusive disease [VOD] etc.) due to complement activation and endothelial damage. Removing the plasma from the product before infusion can eliminate this risk. A second concern is a delayed hemolytic transfusion reaction. The type O donor has B cells that are capable of producing antibody to A or B substance. When these B cells are infused with the graft, they may be stimulated by A or B substance on the recipient's red cells, which can result in a prompt increase in antibody production. A severe hemolytic anemia that can be life-threatening can result 2 to 10 days later. This usually occurs with T-cell depletion of type O donors. Finally, use of plasma from type O donors will add unwanted antibodies (see also major–minor mismatch). In these circumstances one must be careful about the use of both the plasma infusions and the plasma that comes with cellular products.

MAJOR–MINOR MISMATCH

Donor is either A or B and the recipient is the opposite. In this case, there is a risk of both immediate transfusion and infusion of preformed antibody as noted earlier. Thus the product needs to be both RBC and plasma depleted.

Major and minor mismatch stem cell product

Recipient ABO	Donor ABO	Mismatch	Management
O	A, B, AB	Major	Red cell deplete stem cell product
A, B, AB	O	Minor	Plasma deplete stem cell product
A	B	Major–Minor	Both red cell and plasma depletion
B	A	Major–Minor	Both red cell and plasma depletion

Transfusion restrictions are dependent on the ABO type of donor and recipient

Recipient ABO	Donor ABO	Transfusion Restrictions[1]
O Preformed Anti-A and Anti-B	O	None
	A	• Red cell deplete stem cells • O red cell products • A/AB plasma products[2] • A/AB or type O/B washed platelets[2]
	B	• Red cell deplete stem cells • O red cell products • B/ AB plasma products[3] • B/ AB or type O/A washed products[3]
	AB	• Red cell deplete stem cells • O red cell products • AB plasma products[1,2] • AB or type O/A/B washed platelets[2,3]
A Anti-B	A	• A/AB or washed type O/B platelets
	O	• Plasma deplete stem cells • A or O red cell products • A/AB plasma products • A/AB or type O/B washed platelets[2]
	B	• Plasma deplete stem cells and RBCs • O red cell products • AB plasma products • AB or type O/A/B washed platelets[1]
	AB	• Plasma deplete stem cells and RBCs • A or O red cell products • AB plasma products • AB or type O/A/B washed platelets[2,3]

(continued)

Recipient ABO	Donor ABO	Transfusion Restrictions[1]
B *Anti-A*	B	• B/ AB type O/A washed platelets[3]
	O	• Plasma deplete stem cells • B or O red cell products • B/AB plasma products • B/ AB or type O/A washed platelets[3]
	A	• Plasma deplete stem cells and RBCs • B or O red cell products • AB plasma products • AB or type O/A/B washed platelets[2,3]
	AB	• Plasma deplete stem cells and RBCs • B or O red cell products • AB plasma products • AB or type O/A/B washed platelets[2,3]
AB	AB	• AB or type O/A/B washed platelets[2,3]
	O	• Plasma deplete stem cells • O red cell products • AB plasma products • AB or type O/A/B washed platelets[2,3]
	A	• Plasma deplete stem cells • A, B, or O red cell products • AB plasma products • AB or type O/A/B washed platelets[2,3]
	B	• Plasma deplete stem cells • A, B, or O red cell products

Recipient ABO	Donor ABO	Transfusion Restrictions[1]
AB	B	• AB plasma products • AB or type O/A/B washed platelets[2,3]

[1] In situations where the transplant consists of two cord blood products with different ABO/Rh, choose the most conservative transfusion restriction.

[2] Do not want to add more anti A from the product.

[3] Do not want to add more anti B from the product.

Rh AND MINOR RED CELL ANTIGENS

For the most part, these incompatibilities are not associated with acute problems and do not need to be addressed. Rh-negative women receiving Rh-positive cells can be at risk of hemolytic disease of the newborn if their fertility is spared by the transplant. If sparing of fertility in a woman is anticipated, use of red cell-depleted products followed by WinRho is preferred.

REFERENCE

1. Benjamin RJ, Antin JH. ABO-incompatible bone marrow transplantation: The transfusion of incompatible plasma may exacerbate regimen-related toxicity. *Transfusion*. 1999 Nov–Dec;39(11–12):1273–1274.

9. ENGRAFTMENT

Engraftment is defined as an absolute neutrophil (ANC) count greater than 500 cells/μL on two consecutive days or 1,000 cells/μL on one day. Platelet engraftment is defined as an unsupported platelet count greater than 20,000/μL. Recipients of peripheral blood stem cells recover counts faster than recipients of bone marrow. Cord blood tends to be the slowest to engraft. Engraftment can be dependent on the graft-versus-host disease (GVHD) prophylaxis used and is slowest in methotrexate (MTX)-containing regimens.

Transplant	Average Day to Neutrophil Engraftment
Auto-BMT + G-CSF	Day 15–25
Auto-PBSCT + G-CSF	Day 9–12
T-cell depleted allo BMT + GCSF	Day 13–20
Allo-BMT with CNI MTX prophylaxis	Day 22–24
Allo-PBSCT with or without MTX prophylaxis	Day 10–14
Cord Blood 1 unit 2 units	Day +40 and later Day 12–24

BMT, bone marrow transplant; CNI, calcineurin inhibitor (e.g., cyclosporine or tacrolimus); GCSF, granulocyte colony-stimulating factor; PBSCT, peripheral blood stem cell transplantation.

10. PREVENTATIVE CARE

Preventative care will vary on the basis of transplant type, protocol, medications, and pretransplant viral studies.

INFECTION PROPHYLAXIS

Please see Chapter 15 on infectious diseases.

HOSPITAL INFECTION CONTROL

Hospital personnel should follow standard infection control and Center for Disease Control (CDC) guidelines to prevent nosocomial infections. The efficacy of different transplant-specific precautions in preventing nosocomial infections has not been studied. Hand washing continues to be the single most critical and effective procedure for preventing infection. If gloves are utilized, they should be changed between patients. All equipment should be sterilized or disinfected and Environment Protection Agency (EPA) registered.

Allogeneic hematopoietic stem cell transplantation (HSCT) patients should be placed in private rooms that have >12 air exchanges per hour and high-efficiency particulate air filters (HEPA) that are capable of removing particles ≥0.3 μm in diameter. It is generally considered good practice to treat all immunocompromised people in HEPA-filtered rooms although the data are less clear than for allogeneic HSCT.

GUT DECONTAMINATION

Gut decontamination is used in some centers in all myeloablative and cord allogeneic procedures. Its use is most important when the risk of GVHD is higher (i.e., mismatched and URDs). In autologous and T-cell depleted patients an alternative is to use levofloxacin 500 mg PO starting on day 1 and continue through engraftment.

Nonabsorbable antibiotic regimen may include nystatin 2 MU, bacitracin 500 mg, and polymixin 10^6 units orally every 8 hours. Many patients are not able to tolerate these oral medications during transplantation, but if they can take it early in conditioning, the intestinal track tends to stay sterile as long as they are treated in a HEPA environment.

SKIN AND ORAL CARE

HSCT patients should take daily showers or baths. Skin sites that have the potential to be portal sites for infection should be inspected daily. Good dental hygiene before and after HSCT (at least 1 year) is important. All patients should receive a dental evaluation as part of the pretransplant assessment. Dental work including eliminating sources of infection should take place before conditioning therapy.

In addition to gut decontamination, patients should receive mouth care 4 to 6 times/day. Mouth care should start with conditioning and continue through engraftment. Mouth care and daily oral hygiene is encouraged to prevent infection secondary to mucosal breakdown, it does not reduce the incidence of mucositis. Oral rinses should be administered 4 to 6 times/day. Teeth should be brushed with an ultrasoft toothbrush or Toothette twice daily. When platelets are >50 K and ANC >500 patients can resume flossing.

It is important to note that nystatin is often prepared in a sugar-based suspension, which can, over time, promote tooth decay and exacerbate diabetes. It is possible to use nystatin in a water-based formula if desired.

Clotrimazole troches and other azole antifungal medications will affect the levels of cyclosporine, tacrolimus, and sirolimus by increasing the bioavailability.

At the time of discharge, patients should continue to use mouth rinses for at least 2 to 4 weeks. They can resume routine dental cleanings once counts have fully recovered.

Dental Prophylaxis

Standard regimens include:

Amoxicillin 2 g, 1 hour preprocedure
Ampicillin 2 g IV, 30 minutes before procedure

PCN allergy:

Clindamycin 600 mg PO, 1 hour preprocedure
Cephalexin or cefdroxil 2 g PO, 1 hour preprocedure

Azithromycin 500 mg PO, 1 hour pre procedure

Clarithromycin 500 mg PO, 1 hour pre procedure

Common Oral Conditions

Hairy Tongue

Have patients try to increase moisture in their mouth during waking hours. Encourage patients to vigorously brush their tongue with a toothbrush as far back as possible. If no mucositis and ANC >500, it is okay to use firm toothbrush or tongue scraper. Oxygel scrub (glyoxide) or a 1:1 peroxide and water mix can be tried. Oxygel is 11% urea peroxide in a glycerine gel made by Block Drug Co. Jersey City, NJ. Peroxide has a drying effect so it is important to keep the mouth moist.

Xerostomia

Use approaches are as follows:

- Mouthwashes without alcohol only.
- Artificial saliva products such as MouthKote.
- Sugarless gum or hard sour candies (patients should be instructed to use caution since they are prone to caries).
- Biotene mouth products.
- Ensure that patient is getting adequate fluoride. Most patients are drinking bottled water and therefore may not be getting enough.
- Pilocarpine (Salagen) 5 mg PO BID.
- Pilocarpine 1% 15 gtts in water QID. Results are variable.
- Evoxac (Cevilemine) 30 mg TID.

PREVENTING BACTERIAL INTRAVASCULAR CATHETER-RELATED INFECTIONS

Catheter care should follow published guidelines. Caps and dressings should be maintained on a routine basis.

POST-HSCT RESTRICTIONS, REDUCING THE RISK OF INFECTION WHILE AT HOME

Most transplant centers will have specific guidelines for patients to follow. Patients should follow transplant center–specific instructions. The following is a general overview of post-HSCT care.

- Avoid environmental exposures by hand washing frequently. Exposures can occur when preparing food, changing diapers, touching plants or dirt, pet contact, secretion contact.
- Respiratory infections may be prevented if patients observe the following precautions: hand washing, avoid close contact with persons with respiratory illness (if unavoidable the person with illness should wear a mask), avoid crowded/public areas, avoid high-risk occupations, avoid construction sites, damp basements, attics, travel, tobacco exposure, marijuana (associated with invasive fungal infections), gardening, yard work, wood-burning fire places.
- Infections that occur because of direct contact can be minimized by advising patients to avoid the following: contact with soil, plants, animal feces/urine, diapers and others.
- Water safety: HSCT recipients should avoid contact with recreational water to avoid *Cryptosporidium*, *Escherichia. coli O157:H7*, sewage, or animal/human waste. Well water should be avoided if possible. If the well is from a municipal community where the water is tested frequently it may be regarded as safe. HSCT recipients who drink tap water should check their local source often for increase in bacterial levels. Other precautions include avoiding fountain beverages, frozen/fruit drinks, iced tea/coffee and other products made with tap water. Bottled water should be from a distributor that sterilizes the water. Examples of sterile water are Dasani and Aquafina. All carbonated drinks are considered sterile.
- Travel: In general, travel should be avoided for the first 6 to 12 months post HSCT. Any travel in this period should be discussed with the transplant physician.
- Safe sexual precautions: Having intimate contact with a partner may increase the risk for infections but a patient may resume sexual activity when he or she feels ready. Nonintercourse sexual expression (i.e., hugging and kissing) with the significant other is encouraged after transplant. The following are guidelines to help minimize the risk of infections in patients who are in nonmonogamous relationships

or seeking relationships with new individuals after transplantation. The risk of acquiring disease is very low in long-standing monogamous relationships.

- Single partners – partner should not have a cold, flu, or cold sores; platelets should be greater than 50,000; latex condom should be used to reduce the risk of acquisition of cytomegalovirus, herpes simplex virus, and human papilloma virus, as well as other sexually transmitted pathogens. Condom use will also, theoretically, reduce the risk of acquisition of human herpes virus. Data regarding the use and efficacy of "female condoms" are incomplete, but these devices should be considered as a risk-reduction strategy. Patients may receive, but not administer oral sex. Oral exposure to feces should be avoided at all costs to reduce the risk of intestinal infections (e.g., cryptosporidiosis, shigellosis, campylobacteriosis, amebiasis, giardiasis, and hepatitis A and B, E.coli). Anal intercourse should be avoided since the risk of infection is high. Radiation and GVHD cause an increase in dryness in the lining of the vagina. To make intercourse comfortable and to help prevent tearing of the mucosal membrane, water soluble lubricant or gel, which contains no perfume or coloring, is recommended. Some brands include Replens, Astroglide, Lubrin, K-Y Jelly, Surgilube, Today Personal Lubricant, and Ortho Personal Lubricant. Do not use a Vaseline or oil-based lubricant as these may cause an increase in yeast infections.

- Pet Safety: Patients should not routinely part with their pets but in general, minimal contact is recommended. HSCT recipients should avoid contact with animal feces to reduce the risk for toxoplasmosis, cryptosporidiosis, salmonellosis, and campylobacteriosis. HSCT recipients should not clean cages, litter boxes, or dispose of animal waste. Any pet that is ill or has diarrhea should be evaluated by a veterinarian. Contact with reptiles (food or anything the reptile has touched) should be avoided because of the risk of salmonellosis. Direct contact with birds, exotic pets, and fish should be avoided. If avoiding direct contact with pets is not possible, then the HSCT recipient should be advised to wear gloves and wash hands thoroughly.

DIET, EARLY POSTTRANSPLANT, REDUCED BACTERIA

In general, the HSCT diet consists of foods considered to be low in pathogenic bacteria. Dietary restrictions and food safety practices should be reviewed before conditioning begins to ensure that the patient and his/her care givers understand the importance of adherence to the special diet. HSCT patients should not consume any raw or undercooked meat, including beef, poultry, lamb, wild game, or seafood (including oysters and clams). Raw eggs or foods that contain raw eggs should not be consumed. HSCT patients should avoid thin-skinned fruits and vegetables unless cooked until well done.

Following is a general list of foods allowed and not allowed. This may vary per transplant center and geographic location.

Food Category	Foods Permitted	Foods Not Permitted
Beverages	Coffee, tea, cocoa, pasteurized milk and frappes, carbonated beverages, pasteurized juices, canned nutritional supplements, tap water, spring water	Raw milk (unpasteurized) Eggnog or milkshakes made with raw eggs Fresh apple cider
Meat, Fish, Eggs, Poultry	Well cooked: meat, fish, shellfish, eggs, and poultry Canned meats and fish (tuna)	Raw or rare meat, fish, shellfish, eggs, and poultry. Cold cuts from a Deli
Dairy products	Pasteurized milk, lactaid milk, chocolate milk, cream, nondairy creamer, ice cream, sherbet, yogurt, pudding, cottage cheese, cream cheese, American cheese, all cooked pasteurized cheeses	Raw milk (unpasteurized), soft serve ice cream or frozen yogurt, hand-packed ice cream or frozen yogurt. The following cheeses: feta, brie, camembert, queso fresco, blue cheese, gorgonzola, cheeses sliced at a deli, imported cheeses

(*continued*)

Food Category	Foods Permitted	Foods Not Permitted
Breads, cereals, potatoes, rice, pasta, and pastry	All prepackaged breads, muffins, cakes, pies, rolls, donuts, cookies. All boxed hot or cold cereals (except those with dried fruit or nuts) All cooked potatoes, rice, noodles Packaged crackers and snack foods	Bakery breads, cakes, muffins, donuts Cream or custard filled cakes from the refrigerated section Commercially prepared potato or macaroni salad Popcorn (due to dental problems)
Vegetables	All cooked vegetables (wash well and cook thoroughly)	Raw vegetables, salads
Fruits	All cooked or canned fruits, bottled or canned fruit juices, pasteurized fruit juice	All raw fruit and garnishes, unpasteurized fruit juice, dried fruits
Nuts	Processed peanut butter, cooked nuts	Raw nuts, fresh peanut butter
Miscellaneous	Salt, cooked spices, sauces, and gravy, individually packaged ketchup, mustard, mayonnaise, relish, sugar, butter, creamer. Thoroughly cooked frozen dinners, and frozen pizza Canned entrees	Uncooked spices including black pepper, raw honey

LONG-TERM PREVENTION OF INFECTIONS AFTER HSCT – VACCINATIONS

Cellular and humoral immunity are severely depressed after transplantation. Antibody titers to diseases such as tetanus, polio, and others decline, often to levels that may not be protective. Moreover, within the first year after transplantation there may be a suboptimal response to vaccines. Therefore, it is important to administer vaccines after the patient has reconstituted his or her immune system. B- and T-cell function can take 12 months or longer to restore if the patient has GVHD or is still on immunosuppressive medications. Live vaccines should not be utilized, until at least 2 years after HSCT and then only if the patient is no longer on immunosuppression and has no chronic GVHD. The use of varicella vaccine has not been studied after HSCT and is generally not administered.

It is also important to monitor immunoglobulin (Ig) G levels after HSCT and replace gammaglobulin if the patients become hypogammaglobulinemic. The duration of replacement varies pending recovery of active immunity. A convenient schedule is replacement for 6 months followed by reevalation. If IgG levels are maintained, replacement can be stopped. Otherwise, continue monthly intravenous gammaglobulin reevaluating approximately every 6 months. Vaccine or toxoid

	Time post HSCT		
Inactivated vaccine or toxoid	12	14	24
Diphtheria, tetanus, pertussis	DTP[a] or DT[b] or Dt[c]	DTP or DT or Dt	DTP or DT or Dt
Haemophilus influenzae type b (Hib) conjugate	Hib conjugate	Hib conjugate	Hib conjugate
Hepatitis B[d]	Hep B	Hep B	Hep B
7-valent pneumococcal vaccine	PP7	PP7	
23-valent pneumoccal polysaccharide (PPV23)			PPV23
Hepatitis A	Routine administration not indicated		
Influenza	Lifelong, seasonal administration. Begins before HSCT and resumes 6 months after		
Meningococcal	Routine administration not indicated		
Inactivated polio (IPV)	IPV	IPV	IPV

(*continued*)

Live-attenuated vaccine

Measles-mumps-rubella (MMR)		MMR[e]
Varicella vaccine	Contraindicated	

CDC recommendations.[1]

[a] Diphtheria toxoid-tetanus toxoid-pertussis vaccine (DTP).

[b] Diphtheria toxoid-tetanus toxoid (DT). Should be used when there is a contraindication to pertussis.

[c] Tetanus-diphtheria toxoid.

[d] Hep B recommended for adults with known risk factors.

[e] MMR – first dose should be administered 24 months after HSCT if the person is considered immunocompetent. Use of live vaccines is indicated only among immunocompetent persons and is contraindicated for recipients after HSCT who are not presumed immunocompetent.

REFERENCE

1. Guidelines for preventing opportunistic infections among hematopoietic stem cell transplant recipients. *MMWR*. 2000;49:rr-10:1–128.

11. TRANSPLANT-RELATED COMPLICATIONS

When making a differential diagnosis in a patient who has undergone hematopoietic stem cell transplantation (HSCT), it is critical to have a solid understanding of the entire course of treatment. This includes transplant type (autologous or allogeneic) stem cell source (marrow, peripheral blood [PB], or cord blood), donor match (related or unrelated, matched or mismatched), interval post-HSCT (early or late), graft-versus-host disease (GVHD) prophylaxis, infectious prophylaxis, current immune suppressive medications, conditioning regimen (ablative or nonmyeloablative), and length of granulocytopenia. Transplant-related toxicities can include treatment-related organ damage, infection, GVHD, or any other combination. Time course is generally thought of as follows: early – first 30 days when pancytopenia and the direct effect of chemotherapy is the greatest; mid – day 15 to roughly 100; and late – after day 100. There is often an overlap in timing of complications.

In the remainder of the book you will find information on the following transplant-related complications:

GVHD – prevention, acute and chronic
Engraftment syndrome
Infectious disease
Graft rejection and Graft failure
Gastrointestinal complications
Pulmonary complications
Veno-occlusive disease
Special transfusion-related situations
Cardiovascular complications
Neurological complications
Cystitis
Donor lymphocyte infusion

12. GRAFT-VERSUS-HOST DISEASE – PROPHYLAXIS AND ACUTE

OVERVIEW

Graft-versus-host disease (GVHD) is one of the classical complications of allogeneic stem cell transplantation. It is dependent on the presence of histocompatibility differences between the host and the donor. These can be minor antigens in the case of matched transplantation or major histocompatibility complex (MHC) antigens if there is some human leukocyte antigen (HLA) incompatibility. Minor antigens are presented to the T cells presumably in the same way that bacterial or viral antigens are presented to T cells. Thus, in essence, the graft is functioning as if there were a severe infection, and the graft tries to eradicate antigens that are intrinsic to the host. This results in the tissue damage that we clinically recognize as GVHD.

There are two main categories of GVHD, acute and chronic, each with two subcategories:

Classic acute GVHD
Persistent, recurrent, or late-onset acute GVHD
Chronic GVHD
Classic chronic GVHD

Previously, acute GVHD (aGVHD) was arbitrarily assigned to all allogeneic manifestations that occurred before day 100. Similarly cGVHD was the manifestations occurring after day 100. This distinction is no longer considered useful. It is now recognized that there can be late-onset aGVHD (frequently but not exclusively after reduced intensity transplantation) that looks clinically like aGVHD.

Moreover, there can be cGVHD that occurs early after transplantation, which is considered classic without features of aGVHD, and an overlap syndrome in which features of chronic and acute GVHD appear together.

PROPHYLACTIC REGIMENS

Effective prophylaxis is limited by an incomplete understanding of the pathophysiology of the disease. Traditionally, aGVHD

Category	Time of Symptoms After HSCT or DLI	Presence of Acute GVHD Features*	Presence of Chronic GVHD Features*
Acute GVHD			
Classic acute GVHD	≤100 days	Yes	No
Persistent, recurrent, or late-onset acute GVHD	>100 days	Yes	No
Chronic GVHD			
Classic chronic GVHD	No time limit	No	Yes
Overlap syndrome	No time limit	Yes	Yes

DLI, donor lymphocyte infusion. GVHD, graft-versus-host disease; HSCT, hematopoietic stem cell transplantation.

Filipovich AH, Weisdorf D, Pavletic S, et al. National Institutes of Health consensus disease I. Diagnosis and staging working group report. *Biol Blood marrow Transplant.* 2005;11(12):945–956.

is thought to be the most critical risk factor; therefore, the focus has been to prolong or intensify aGVHD prophylaxis to reduce the incidence of cGVHD. Prolonging the immune suppression has mixed results. Drugs are often used in combination in an attempt to block several pathways thought to cause GVHD. Use of calcineurin inhibitors in conjunction with methotrexate is the most common combined regimen. Institutions use a variety of combinations. See section on each agent for dose and toxicity.

1. Tacrolimus/methotrexate (MTX) or cyclosporine/MTX superior to single-agent prophylaxis. When calcineurin inhibitors are used with lower doses of MTX, so-called mini methotrexate may attenuate mucositis caused by MTX.
2. Tacrolimus/mycophenolate mofetil (MMF) or cyclosporine/MMF. MMF is an alternative for patients who are unable to take MTX.
3. Sirolimus/tacrolimus/MTX or sirolimus/tacrolimus may allow for lower doses or the elimination of MTX.

AGENTS USED FOR PROPHYLAXIS

Methotrexate

Mechanism of Action

Blocks the enzyme dihydrofolate reductase, which inhibits the conversion of folic acid to tetrahydrofolic acid, resulting in an inhibition of the key precursors of DNA, RNA, and cellular protein.

Metabolism

It is bound to serum albumin. Hepatic and intracellular metabolism. Half-life is 2 hours; 50 to 100% is renally excreted. Peak concentration is 3 to 12 hours after administration.

Dose

For GVHD prophylaxis (when combined with tacrolimus only): MTX 15 mg/m^2 on day + 1, followed by 10 mg/m^2 on days 3, 6, and 11. At Dana-Farber, if used with tacrolimus and rapamycin, it is given on days 1, 3, and 6 only (not day 11) and the dose is decreased to 5 mg/m^2 (mini-MTX dosing).

These doses are too low for MTX levels to be of use. Studies demonstrate that skipping doses is associated with an increased risk of GVHD. Therefore, efforts to administer MTX while minimizing toxicity are warranted. Recent studies suggest that doses as low as 5 mg/m^2 are effective. Redundant

Toxicity

It is important to assess patient for pleura or pericardial effusions, ascites, third-spacing or renal failure before each dose. MTX will exacerbate chemotherapy-induced mucositis and it may be necessary to hold or reduce the dose of MTX if there is airway compromise secondary to mucositis.

Methotrexate/Leucovorin Rescue Recommendations

It has been noted that certain patients receiving MTX for GVHD prophylaxis may be at higher risk for MTX-related toxicities including oral mucositis and possibly hepatic veno-occlusive disease (VOD). Neville et al. (1992)[1] suggest that the use of leucovorin rescue may reduce these toxicities attributable to MTX and might allow accelerated engraftment as well without compromise in the MTX immunoprophylaxis against GVHD. (Note: This small study may have missed any compromise in effectiveness of GVHD prophylaxis.)

Patients believed to be at greatest risk for MTX-related toxicities (i.e., late engraftment, hepatic dysfunction, severe mucositis) are those with either decreased renal function (serum creatinine > 1.5 X baseline or > 2.0 mg/dL) or significant fluid collections, that is, ascites, pleural effusions, and so on where MTX can accumulate and thus delay MTX clearance. Hyperbilirubinemia is not an indication for leucovorin therapy, and leucovorin therapy is not indicated if the risk has resolved (e.g., creatinine level has improved or fluid collection has resolved).

Leucovorin rescue schema for patients with the high-risk features mentioned are as follows:

- Twelve hours after day +1 MTX (15 mg/m^2), give leucovorin 15 mg/m^2 intravenous (IV) every 6 hours for three doses (max single dose = 30 mg)
- Twelve hours after day +3 MTX (10 mg/m^2), give leucovorin 10 mg/m^2 IV every 6 hours for six doses (max dose = 25 mg/m^2)
- Twenty four hours after subsequent doses of MTX, give leucovorin 10 mg/m^2 IV every 6 hours for eight doses (max dose = 25 mg/m^2)

Note: If leucovorin is given, MTX levels should not be measured.

Calcineurin Inhibitors Tacrolimus and Cyclosporine
Both tacrolimus and cyclosporine (CSA) have a similar mechanism of action and toxicity. Tacrolimus is slightly more potent and has a more reliable area under the curve (AUC).

Mechanism of Action
Cyclosporine binds to cyclophyllin and tacrolimus binds to FKBP12. In either case, the complex inhibits calcineurin phosphatase. Calcineurin is a protein necessary for a number of cellular processes and calcium-dependent signal transduction pathways. These drugs inhibit activation and proliferation of T-lymphocytes by interfering with interleukin (IL)-2 production, and expression of IL-2 receptor. They interfere with cell cycle in G0 phase.

Tacrolimus (Prograf, FK-506)

- Metabolism: CYP450–3A4 system in the liver and intestine. Ninety-two percent is excreted in bile. Absorption is decreased with food. Peak level varies when the drug is administered orally (1.5 to 3.5 hours), IV 1 to 2 hours. Half-life is 21 to 61 hours in healthy volunteers. Average half-life is 18 hours in HSCT patients. Half-life is prolonged with hepatic dysfunction.

■ Dose: 0.02 to 0.05 mg/kg IV (continuous over 24 hours). It is convenient to start on day –3 and continue until the patient is able to take oral medication. The IV to oral conversion can be approximated as the IVCI daily dose × 3, divided into two doses/day. Levels need to be followed daily until they are stable. Standard oral dose used is 0.05 mg/kg every 12 hours rounded to the nearest 0.5 mg. Patients may require a lesser dose to maintain therapeutic levels depending on albumin levels and hematocrit. Drugs that alter P450 metabolism may increase or decrease levels of tacrolimus. Schedule and therapeutic levels will vary by protocol and institution. Levels of 5 to 10 ng/mL seem to be better tolerated in HSCT patients than higher levels. Note: Spuriously high levels will often be obtained if drawn from the line used for infusion of the drug. Confirm unsuspected or abnormally high levels with the level drawn from periphery.

■ Dose adjustments are based on clinical toxicity, blood levels, and GVHD. For supratherapeutic levels (between 10 and 15), the dose is decreased by 25% every 2 days. If level is >15 hold the dose until level drops to <10 and restart dose at 25% dose reduction. If level is <5, dose may be increased by 25%. Once levels are therapeutic, measure as clinically indicated. The dose of tacrolimus should be tapered beginning week 9 if there is no evidence of active GVHD. The drug can be reduced slowly and intermittently in increments allowed by capsule size. Since doses are individualized, the taper needs to be individualized as well. Tacrolimus should be eliminated on week 26 if clinically feasible. If GVHD is present, the tapering schedule will be determined by the treating transplant physician according to the patient's clinical condition. Taper schedule may vary by protocol and institute. If a patient has GVHD, the tacrolimus should not be tapered until the GVHD has been controlled for 1 month.

Cyclosporine

Dose and schedule should be determined by protocol. In general:

■ Dose is 2.5 mg/kg IV every 12 hours (given over 2 to 4 hours) until the patient is able to take orally. Convert to oral as soon as clinically feasible. IV conversion to oral is 1:3 to 4.

Neoral/Gengraf (cyclosporine, modified emulsion) has better bioavailability than sandimmune. There is some data to suggest the conversion of IV to PO is 1:1 with neoral/gengraf versus 1:3 to 4 with sandimmune; however, the manufacturer suggests using the same IV/PO conversion factor for both formulations and titrate according to the level. It is important when writing prescriptions to specify neoral/gengraf or sandimmune with "No Substitutions." Changing preparation may result in a sudden increase in absorption, levels, and toxicity.

- Standard PO dose is 5 mg/kg/dose every 12 hours.
- Trough levels should be monitored. Check the level after three doses have been administered. In general, levels of 200 to 400 are acceptable but may vary with protocol and institute. Dose modifications are made primarily on the basis of clinical response (i.e., GVHD control and toxicity). Note: CSA will have spurious high levels if drawn from the line used for infusion of the drug. Confirm unsuspected or abnormally high levels with level drawn from periphery.
- A taper can begin around day 50 to 60 if there are no signs of GVHD (vary by protocol and institute). Adults taking capsules can decrease the dose by 25 mg/week (e.g., 600 mg every 12 hours $\times$ 1 week; 600 mg A.M., 575 mg P.M., second week; 575 every 12 hours third week). Cyclosporine should not be tapered until GVHD has been controlled for at least 1 month.

Common Toxicity of Calcineurin Inhibitors

There is no strict correlation between toxicity and serum levels. Ensure adequate hydration and magnesium supplementation. Be alert to the use of other nephrotoxins and drug interactions (especially inhibition or activation of hepatic P450 systems). Avoid aminoglycosides if possible. If changing between CSA and tacrolimus, the original agent must be discontinued for 24 hours before starting the other agent.

CARDIOVASCULAR TOXICITY

HYPERTENSION

If calcineurin induced, treat with β-blocker or calcium-channel blocker (nifedipine or amlodipine are recommended). Avoid diltiazem/verapamil if possible because of the potent P450 inhibition causing increased levels of tacrolimus or CSA.

Hydralazine does not seem to be as effective. Prazocin or tora-zocin may also be used. ACE or ATII inhibitors can be used if renal function is carefully monitored to prevent exacerbation of reduced renal blood flow caused by calcineurin inhibitors. Calcineurin inhibitors cause renal afferent arteriole vasoconstriction. Be cautious with patients who have hypertension and are thrombocytopenic.

THROMBOTIC MICROANGIOPATHY OR TRANSPLANT-ASSOCIATED MICROANGIOPATHY

Calcineurin inhibitors may cause thrombotic microangiopathy. This is often referred to as TTP or HUS, but it is pathophysiologically distinct from those diseases. It is presumably due to renal afferent arteriolar spasm and red blood cell injury as they are forced through a small space. It often responds to reduction in calcineurin inhibitor dose. It does not typically respond to plasmapheresis. One may anticipate an approximately 5% to 10% rate of TMA. If the patient recieves the combination of tacrolimus and sirolimus, the incidence may be higher. Importantly, it responds to a reduction or discontinuation of tacrolimus dose rather than that of sirolimus. Attempt to keep tacrolimus at the low end of the therapeutic range. Monitor hematocrit, platelets, LDH, and creatinine. Clinical diagnosis is established by hemolysis and evidence of microangiopathy.

High plasma triglycerides may decrease free CSA/tacrolimus while not altering whole blood levels. Low plasma triglyceride may increase availability and thereby increase the efficacy and toxicity without altering blood levels.

Renal Toxicity

Close monitoring of creatinine and dose adjustments are recommended if the creatinine rises. CSA/tacrolimus can cause increased uric acid levels. If levels are in the upper end of the normal range and the creatinine is elevated you should adjust the dose. Hydrate aggressively and avoid other nephrotoxins when possible. It is important not to wait for level or marked increase in creatinine to adjust dosing.

Neurologic Toxicity

Neurologic toxicity includes tremors (common), ataxia, paresthesias, seizures (check calcium and magnesium levels as well as CSA/tacrolimus level), somnolence, cortical blindness,

Creatinine	Adjustment
↑ > 2 × baseline	Check level the same day
↑ > 2 × baseline × 48 hours	Reduce dose by 25%
Creatinine > 2.0 mg/dL	Hold one dose and recheck creatinine level in 12 hours. If creatinine level is stable or ↓ give dose at 75% of daily dose. If creatinine level is rising, continue to hold and recheck creatinine every 12 hours. Once creatinine < 1.8 mg/dL or < 1.5 × baseline, attempt to reintroduce CSA/ tacrolimus back toward the scheduled every 12 hours dosing. Attempt to increase the dose back to targeted dose every 48 hours. Adjust other nephrotoxins as appropriate

If the patient is hypotensive or septic then hold one dose that day to avoid further damage.

and nightmares/hallucinations. Jitteriness and paresthesias do not require a dose alteration. If the level is high, aim for the lower end of therapeutic range and monitor. Replete calcium and magnesium daily. If a seizure or cortical blindness occurs, optimize blood pressure, stabilize CSA/tacrolimus levels and aim for lower levels of therapeutic range. Obtain brain magnetic resonance imaging (MRI), looking for posterior leukoencephalopathy (reversible if induced by calcineurin inhibitors).

A burning sensation in hands and feet in the absence of rash may occur during IV infusion, this is thought to be a reaction to the Cremophore diluent. If this occurs, slow the infusion. If it does not resolve and patient can tolerate oral therapy, consider changing to oral administration.

Electrolyte Abnormalities
Decreased magnesium and increased potassium levels are common.

Endocrine Toxicity
DIABETES
Calcineurin inhibitors cause insulin resistance. Additional elevation of blood sugar is likely when used with corticosteroids.

HEPATIC DYSFUNCTION HYPERBILIRUBINEMIA
Tacrolimus /Sirolimus is implicated less than cyclosporine.

Other Effects
Gingival hyperplasia and hypertrichosis are seen with CSA and not tacrolimus.

Drug Interactions with Calcineurin Inhibitors and Sirolimus
Levels of CSA, tacrolimus, and Sirolimus increase when the hepatic P450 system is inhibited.

Levels of CSA, tacrolimus, and Sirolimus decrease with the hepatic P450 system is induced.

Common CSA, tacrolimus and sirolimus drug interactions.

Antifungals	Tacrolimus(%)	Sirolimus (%)
Voriconazole	66 reduction	90 reduction
Posaconazole	33–50 reduction	33 reduction
Fluconazole (slow inhibitor)	33–50 reduction	33 reduction

For patients with renal impairment, weigh the relative importance of the drug versus the risk of additional nephrotoxins.

Approximate dose adjustments for azole antifungals:

Mycophenolate Mofetil (MMF, CellCept)

Mechanism of Action
Inhibits IMP dehydrogenase, which blocks nucleic acid synthesis and inhibits lymphocyte proliferation. Limited data suggests that it can successfully replace MTX for GVHD prophylaxis. It may be useful in patients with effusions and/or hepatic or renal failure and who are unable to receive methotrexate.

Metabolism
There is 94% bioavailability. MMF is a prodrug which is hydrolyzed to mycophenolic acid, the active metabolite in the liver. MMF is renally eliminated as the inactive metabolite, mycophenolic acid glucuronide (MPAG). MPAG is not dialyzable and accumulates in renal failure but the toxicity is unknown.

Tacrolimus inhibitors
Level is increased

- Voriconazole
- Clotrimazole
- Ketoconazole
- Itraconazole
- Fluconazole
- Metronidazole
- Posaconazole
- Erythromycin
- Clarithromycin
- Metoclopramide

- Methylprednisolone
- Nefazodone
- HIV protease inhibitors
- Grapefruit Juice
- Qinupristin/ Dalforpristin
- Verapamil
- Diltiazem
- Ethinyl estradiol
- Norethindrone

Tacrolimus inducers
Level is decreased

- Butalbital
- Carbamazepine
- Caspofungin
- Dexamethasone
- Prednisolone
- Phenobarbital
- Phenytoin
- Rifabutin, Rifampin
- St. John's Wort

Sirolimus inhibitors
Level is increased

- Voriconazole
- Clotrimazole
- Ketoconazole
- Itraconazole
- Fluconazole
- Metronidazole
- Posaconazole
- Micafungin**
- Erythromycin
- Clarithromycin

- Methylprednisolone
- Cyclosporine
- Metoclopramide
- Nefazodone
- HIV protease inhibitors
- Grapefruit Juice
- Qinupristin/Dalforpristin
- Verapamil
- Diltiazem
- Ethinyl estradiol
- Norethindrone

**A 20% increase in level is predicted. In our experience this is inconsistent. We do not empirically reduce the dose. We follow levels and adjust as necessary.

Sirolimus inducers
Level is decreased

- Butalbital
- Carbamazepine
- Dexamethasone
- Prednisolone
- Phenobarbital
- Phenytoin
- Rifabutin
- Rifampin
- St. John's Wort

Dose
Dose is 15 mg/kg actual body weight (maximum 1,000 to 1,500 mg/dose) TID or BID IV or oral. No adjustments are needed for hepatic failure. No adjustments necessary for renal insufficiency unless patient is on dialysis. If dialysis is needed, MMF dose may be reduced to 25% to 50% of the starting dose. There should be a gap of at least 2 hours between antacids and MMF because of decreased absorption due to the antacids.

Side Effects
Include GI (nausea, vomiting, diarrhea) and mild to moderate bone marrow suppression.

Sirolimus (Rapamycin, Rapamune)

Mechanism of Action
Like tacrolimus, sirolimus binds to FKBP12. However, this complex inhibits mTOR rather than calcineurin. mTOR is centrally situated in cellular response to stress, and its inhibition results in a reduction of several cellular processes including transcription and translation. Sirolimus inhibits T cells in the G1 phase of mitosis.

Metabolism
Primarily metabolized by hepatic and intestinal P450 enzymes. Half-life is approximately 60 hours.

Dose
The loading dose 12 mg followed by 4 mg daily. A reasonable guideline is to aim for levels between 3 and 12 ng/mL. Therapeutic levels may vary by institution and protocol. A taper of 1/3 every 9 weeks should begin around day 50 to 60 if there is no evidence of GVHD.

Toxicity
Hyperlipidemia and/or hypertriglyceridemia is common and may require therapy with a statin. Cytopenias and mild neutropenia/thrombocytopenia may also occur. Sirolimus may contribute to TMA when used in conjunction with tacrolimus. There is no intrinsic renal or neurotoxicity, which makes it a good agent to combine with tacrolimus.

Drug interactions of sirolimus are the same as those of calcineurin inhibitors. Also of note is the strong drug interaction when used with voriconazole. If used together, decrease the sirolimus dose by 90%, and monitor levels.

Antithymocyte Globulin

There are two forms of antithymocyte globulin (ATG) that are commonly used. ATGAM is produced in horses and is typically administered at 40 mg/kg/day for 4 days. Thymoglobulin is produced in rabbits. Dosing is less standard but 1.5 mg/kg/day for 4 days is commonly used. Both are administered over 6 to 12 hours to avoid infusional toxicity and reduce allergic reactions. It is used as prophylaxis for GVHD in some regimens and as part of conditioning in aplastic anemia.

Toxicity

Toxicities include anaphylaxis (have epinephrine 0.3 cc of 1:1,000 at bedside given SQ in the event of a reaction), fever, chills, rash, joint pain (serum sickness), and renal toxicity and may also cause myelosuppression. ATG may predispose to Epstein-Barr virus (EBV) lymphoproliferative disorders.

Alemtuzumab (Campath)

This is an antiCD52 monoclonal antibody that is used in some reduced intensity regimens. Dose can be 40 to 60 mg/day given on days –2 and –1. It also has infusional toxicity and results in in vivo T-cell depletion that may reduce the GVL effect resulting in higher relapse rates and increased susceptibility to infection. Usually its use requires DLI subsequently.[2]

Donor T-Cell Depletion

The approach of T-cell depletion (TCD) relies primarily on the removal of putative effector cells of GVHD from the donor graft before transplantation. There are multiple methods to TCD. Methods of TCD include pan-T-cell monoclonal antibody (MoAB) + complement, selective T-cell MoAB + complement, MoAB + magnetic beads, counterflow centrifugal elutriation, soybean lectin agglutination + elutriation, MoAB–immunotoxin conjugate, positive selection of CD34-expressing cells, and others. These methods differ in the number of T cells removed (1.5 to 4 logs), the extent of removal of natural killer (NK) cells, monocytes, and myeloid progenitors, and the requirement for prophylactic GVHD agents.

T-cell depletion may be used in combination with other GVHD prophylactic agents such as calcineurin inhibitors, sirolimus, and/or MTX.

The overall success of TCD depends on whether the reduction in transplant-related mortality outweighs the increase in disease relapse. Potential ways to decrease transplant-related relapse rates after TCD include selective TCD, for example, CD8 depletion, intensify ablation regimen, post HSCT immune modulation, cytokines (IL-2) and donor T-cell infusion post-HSCT. Results of TCD studies vary depending on the method used.

ACUTE GVHD

Acute GVHD occurs when donor T cells recognize host antigens as foreign, resulting in T-cell lymphocyte stimulation (antigen presentation, T-cell activation and T-cell proliferation) and T-cell and secondary effector cell response (cytokine secretion, cytotoxic T cells, NK cells). Contribution of specific subsets remains uncertain. In murine systems, NK cells play a role in GVHD development. The development of aGVHD may be triggered by the initial tissue damage from the conditioning regimen, which releases inflammatory cytokines such as γ-interferon, IL-1, and tumor necrosis factor (TNF). Risk factors for aGVHD include disparity at Class I or Class II HLA loci, female donor $\rightarrow$ male recipient, older patient age, older donor age, multiparous female donor, herpes simplex virus (HSV) or cytomegalovirus (CMV) seropositivity. Patients who develop aGVHD are at higher risk for developing cGVHD.

As noted earlier, aGVHD can be classic, acute, or persistent/recurrent/late. Acute GVHD is characterized by skin, alimentary tract, and/or hepatic involvement.

Classic symptoms include maculopapular rash, nausea, vomiting, anorexia, profuse diarrhea, abdominal cramps, and ileus or cholestatic hepatitis and occur within 100 days of transplantation or DLI. Persistent/recurrent/late aGVHD include features of classic aGVHD (without cGVHD) occurring beyond 100 days post transplantation or DLI. Biopsy is often obtained to support the diagnosis.

Timing

Skin rash typically appears from day +5 to day +50 (or later) with a median time onset at day 20. In nonmyeloablative transplants, onset may occur later. Liver abnormalities often follow within several days. GI involvement is usually seen in the context of skin and liver GVHD but not always. Each organ can be involved in isolation or with any combination of the other two organs.

Histopathology

■ Skin – biopsy is useful when unclear as to whether etiology of the skin rash is due to GVHD or drug eruption. Epidermal abnormalities are most common, with basal cell vacuolar degeneration, eosinophilic "mummified" keratinocytes, and separation of epidermal/dermal junction in severest cases.

■ GI – upper endoscopy is useful in patients with persistent nausea, vomiting, bloating, and/or anorexia. Diagnosis is made by the presence of apoptotic cells in crypts of GI mucosa.

  Colonoscopy/rectal biopsy is useful in patients with diarrhea, and/or who are unresponsive to antidiarrheal agents. It is important to send samples for culture, especially viral (e.g., CMV, adenovirus, HSV). In addition to biopsy, stool studies should be done to further rule out infection.

■ Liver – biopsy may be useful when the etiology is unclear, that is, whether liver function test abnormalities are because of GVHD or other etiologies: hepatic veno-occlusive disease (VOD)/sinusoidal obstructive syndrome (SOS), infection or drug reaction. Biopsy is often performed via transjugular route especially if the patient has low platelet count or other bleeding risk. It is important to request multiple cores to be sent for evaluation to ensure that portal triad/ducts are present in pathology specimens. Biopsy can show focal portal inflammation with bile ductile obliterations. If VOD/SOS is in the differential, transhepatic wedge pressure measurements should be requested as part of the transjugular biopsy procedure (see VOD/SOS).

Staging

Acute GVHD is usually graded according to the modified Glucksberg Scale in which the affected organ is staged individually and an overall grade is assigned on the basis of the severity of each organ system. Most published studies have utilized the Glucksberg scale (or variant thereof) to report aGVHD. Less commonly, the severity of GVHD may also be assessed using the IBMTR Severity Index, which assigns severity on an A–D scale. This scale is similar in its organ staging. Some researchers feel this staging system shows better predictive ability for outcomes. Each system has some advantages. The scheme encompasses all possible combinations of organ stages without overlap.

Staging of Acute GVHD "Modified Glucksberg Scale"

Relative risk of transplant-related mortality and risk of treatment failure (includes nonrelapse mortality and relapse) appears to correlate with GVHD staging.

Extent of Organ Involvement

	Skin	Liver	Gut
Stage			
I	Maculopapular rash on <25% of skin. No associated symptoms	Bilirubin 2–3 mg/dL	Diarrhea 500–1000 mL/day or persistent nausea
II	Rash on 25–50% of skin w/pruritis or other associated symptoms	Bilirubin 3–6 mg/dL	Diarrhea 1,000–1,500 mL/day +/−nausea/vomiting
III	Macular, papular or vesicular eruption with bullous formation or desquamation on >50% of skin	Bilirubin 6–15 mg/dL	Diarrhea 1,500–2,000 mL/day
IV	Generalized erythroderma with bulla formation	Bilirubin > 15 mg/dL	Severe abdominal pain with or without ileus/bleeding or >2 L of stool daily
Grade			
I	Stage 1–2	None	None
II	Stage 3 or	Stage 1 or	Stage 1
III	–	Stage 2–3 or	Stage 2–4
IV	Stage 4 or	Stage 4	–

IBMTR Severity Index

Grade	Skin	Liver	Gut
A	Stage 1	Stage 0	Stage 0
B	Stage 2 or	Stage 1 or 2 or	Stage 1 or 2
C	any organ stage 3		
D	any organ stage 4		

Treatment Guidelines for Acute Graft-versus-Host Disease

Primary Therapy

STEROIDS +/– CALCINEURIN INHIBITOR

All other therapies are investigational at this time and there is no comparative data available.

- Therapy is effective 30 to 60% of the time.
- Typically, therapy needs to be maintained until manifestations are completely resolved; however, be careful of the risk of opportunistic infections and EBV lymphoproliferative disorders that are associated with increased immunosuppression.
- If GVHD develops after TCD CSA or tacrolimus are useful additions.

STEROIDS

Methylprednisolone 0.5 to 2 mg/kg/day. Most common dose is 1 to 2 mg/kg day in grade II to IV GVHD.

- Conversion: Hydrocortisone (1×), Prednisone (4×), Solumedrol (5×), Decadron (20×). In other words, solumedrol to prednisone conversion is 5/4 solumedrol dose.
- There is no standard method to taper steroids once symptoms improve. A reasonable approach is to taper steroids by 10% of original dose per week in the absence of GVHD symptoms and after GVHD has been controlled for about 1 month.

Side effects of steroid therapy include new onset hyperglycemia or exacerbation in diabetic patients, insomnia, increased appetite, psychosis/mania (rare), fluid retension (less likely when using decadron – less minerlocorticoid effect), cushingoid changes, and muscle wasting/weakness.

Topical therapy such as steroids and/or calcineurin inhibitor preparations may be helpful in mild skin GVHD and may allow for lower doses or avoidance of systemic steroid therapy. These medications can be used in combination with antipruritic agents.

TOPICAL STEROIDS

- Desonide 0.05% applied BID to affected area.
- Triamcinolone 0.1% applied BID to affected area. Cannot be used on the face, groin, or axilla.
- Fluocinonide 0.5% applied BID to affected area. Cannot be used on face, groin, or axilla.
- Clobetasol 0.05% applied BID to affected area. Cannot be used on face, groin, or axilla. Most potent and is not recommended for use for longer than 2 weeks.

TOPICAL CALCINEURIN INHIBITORS

- Tacrolimus 0.03% or 0.1% applied BID to affected area.
- Pimecrolimus 1% applied BID to affected area.

Secondary Therapy – Steroid Refractory

Mycophenolate mofetil (CellCept)(described in the section on prophylactic regimen). Mycophenolate mofetil is a very useful adjunct to steroids. Typical dose is 15 mg/kg every 12 hours; may need to start low and work up the dose, for example, 250 mg every 12 hours orally → 1,000 mg every 12 hours orally to manage GI side effects. An advantage is that is can be given orally or IV.

May depress counts, cause GI upset (abdominal discomfort or diarrhea), and cause herpes virus flares. It may interfere with the interpretation of a rectal biopsy. MMF-induced injury mimics GVHD injury.[3]

Tacrolimus or Cyclosporine (Described in Prophylactic Regimen Section)

Tacrolimus or Cyclosporine is used alone or in combination.

ATG [4]

- Horse antithymocyte globulin (ATGAM, Upjohn).
  - Dose for GVHD: 15 to 20 mg/kg/day for 5 to 7 days (after test dose, see subsequent text).
- Rabbit antithymocyte globulin (Thymoglobulin, Sangstat).
  - Reasonable dose is 1.5 mg/kg per day $\times$ 4 days. May be repeated once at 7 to 14 days.

- Specific ATG toxicities:
  - Anaphylaxis
  - Fevers, chills
  - Rash
  - Joint pain (serum sickness)
  - Renal damage
  - May decrease counts
  - Reversible hepatic dysfunction

Denileukin diftitox Ontak (Diphtheria Toxin Conjugated IL-2)

This is a recombinant fusion protein with selective cytotoxicity against activated T lymphocytes based on preferential binding to IL-2 receptors. It has been found to have significant activity against steroid refractory GVHD.

- Phase II data – 70% response rate, 40% CR.
- Phase II dose – 9 μg/kg QD IV days 1, 3, 5, 15, 17, 19.
- Dose-limiting toxicity is transaminitis. Usually transient and peaks about 1 week after administration. There is no dose adjustment needed for renal or hepatic dysfunction.
- Common side effects include the following:
  - Infusional reactions that may be prevented with appropriate premedication using steroids (can use daily steroid dose for GVHD 30 to 60 minutes before infusion), Tylenol, and diphenhydramine. First dose should be administered over 60 minutes, subsequent doses over 30 minutes if there is no reaction.
- Vascular leak syndrome that may present as hypotension (usually during the first 24 hours after infusion), shortness of breath (pulmonary edema), and increasing peripheral edema. Studies suggest that incidence of vascular leak syndrome is reduced when corticosteroids are given as premedication. Leak syndrome is usually associated with low serum albumin. Salt-poor albumin (SPA) infusions should be considered in patients with severe hypoalbuminemia (albumin <2/5) to reduce vascular leak.

Infliximab (Remicade) Monoclonal AntiTNF-α Antibody

Dose includes 5 mg/kg every week but is not well established. Patient must be on antifungal prophylaxis.

Etanercept (Enbrel)

Recombinent DNA–derived protein composed of tumor necrosis receptor (TNR) cloned to the Fc portion of human immunoglobulin (Ig)G1. It binds to TNF-α and blocks its interaction with target cell surface receptors. There is limited phase II data suggestive of activity in primary treatment of aGVHD.

■ Dose is 25 mg SC twice a week (dosing must be at least 72 hours apart). No dose adjustment is necessary for renal or hepatic impairment.

■ Toxicity involves injection site reaction/swelling.

Pentostatin (Nipent)

Inhibits adenosine deaminase, inducing lymphocyte apoptosis. Has activity in steroid refractory GVHD.[5]

■ Maximum tolerated dose in a phase I trial was 1.5 mg/m^2 on days 1 to 3. This may be repeated on day 15 to 17 if necessary.

■ Dose adjustment is needed for renal insufficiency. For a calculated creatinine clearance of 30 to 50 mL/min, dose should be reduced by 50% or 0.75 mg/m^2/day. If creatinine clearance is <30 mL/min Pentostatin should not be used.

■ Dose-limiting toxicity is infection due to lymphopenia (neutrophil count is generally unaffected). Modest liver function test abnormalities and thrombocytopenia have been reported.

■ Phase I data: 63% CR, 13% PR. Future studies are needed.

Extracorporeal Photopheresis (Cutaneous Manifestation Only)

There is limited efficacy data in steroid refractory aGVHD. It is more commonly used in cGVHD (see cGVHD for more details).

Other Therapy

ZENAPAX (DACLIZUMAB)

■ Humanized anti–IL-2 receptor antibody.

■ Studies: increased mortality if used in primary therapy.[6]

■ Dose for GVHD: 1.0 mg/kg daily – usually given every other or every 3rd day for 2 to 3 doses.

■ Specific toxicities: chills, diaphoresis.

ADJUNCTIVE THEARPY
- Oral nonabsorbed steroids (GI GVHD only).
- Budesonide (Entocort) (70% reported response rate) 3 mg orally TID or 9 mg orally daily.

OCTREOTIDE
- May be helpful with diarrhea.
- Start with 500 µg IV every 8 hours. Should respond within 7 days.
- May need to be dose-reduced in some patients.

CHOLESTYRAMINE
Some cases of ileal GVHD may prevent bile acid absorption and contribute to diarrhea.

- Bile acid binders may limit this, but be careful because it may effect the absorption of other drugs.

DIET
It is important to alter diet when making the diagnosis of GI GVHD and once the diagnosis is confirmed. A suggested dietary approach to diarrhea is shown in the subsequent text. It is generally reserved for patients having moderate-to-severe diarrhea. The phase of the diet refers to patient symptoms and guides the clinician as to which stage diet should be followed. Progression of diet occurs as symptoms improve.

GRAFT-VERSES-HOST DISEASE OF THE GUT

Diet Advancement – Phase (Guided by Symptoms)

Phase I
SYMPTOMS
- cramping
- voluminous diarrhea (>1L)
- nausea
- emesis

DIET
- NPO for bowel rest
- TPN with increased calorie and protein provision (35 kcal/kg and 1.8 g/kg) to meet caloric, protein, and vitamin needs.

Phase II

SYMPTOMS

- diarrhea volume decreasing
- forming of stool
- significantly less to no cramping
- no emesis

DIET

- Continue TPN.
- Start clear, isotonic, low residue beverages (Gatorade, diluted juices, Pedialyte, decaffeinated tea, chicken broth, sugar free Jell-O).

Diet must be tolerated for a minimum of 2 to 5 days before progressing to *Phase III*. If liquids are not tolerated (increased cramping, diarrhea, or vomiting), return to *Phase I* for bowel rest. Do not advance from Phase I until stool is formed and cramps markedly improved.

Phase III

SYMPTOMS

- stool is formed (pudding like)
- no emesis
- decreasing diarrhea frequency and volume
- tolerating Phase II diet without complications

DIET

- Continue TPN.
- Progress to solid foods (GVHD stage I diet).
- Limit fat intake (~20 gm/day), lactose free, low insoluble fiber, free of gastric irritants, high soluble fiber (white bread, potato, saltines, cream of wheat, pasta, white rice, canned fruits, Lactaid milk, plain egg, plain tuna and chicken, cooked carrots).

If tolerating all foods with minimal changes in symptoms, progress to *Phase IV*.

Phase III diet is limited in protein due to the limitation of fiber, lactose, and fat. Patients going home tolerating the GVHD stage I diet require supplements or TPN to meet caloric and protein needs.

Phase IV

SYMPTOMS

- formed stool
- minimal cramping
- tolerating >50% of nutritional needs orally

DIET

- Wean TPN as oral intake increases.
- Continue to expand diet (GVHD stage II) adding more starches, protein, and fatty foods.
- Trial standard and high protein supplements such as Boost and Ensure. If diarrhea or cramping increases, remove most recently introduced foods.

Phase V

SYMPTOMS

- no GI cramping
- normal stool
- normal transit time

DIET

- Discontinue TPN.
- Advance diet to regular by adding back 1 new food per day (such as lactose containing products, i.e., yogurt) and assess tolerance.

REFERENCES

1. Nevill TJ, Tirgan MH, Deeg HJ, et al. Influence of post-methotrexate folinic acid rescue on regimen-related toxicity and graft-versus-host disease after allogeneic bone marrow transplantation. *Bone Marrow Transplant.* 1992 May;9(5):349–354.
2. Delgado J, Thompson K, Russell N, et al. Results of alemtuzumab-based reduced-intensity allogeneic transplantation for chronic lymphocytic leukemia: A British Society of Blood and Marrow Transplantation. *Blood.* 2006;107:1724–1730.
3. Basara N, Blau WI, Romer E, et al. Mycophenolate mofetil for the treatment of acute and chronic GVHD in bone marrow transplant patients. *Bone Marrow Transplant.* 1998;22:61–65.
4. MacMillan ML, Weisdorf DJ, Davies SM, et al. Early antithymocyte globulin therapy improves survival in patients with

stetoid-resistant acute graft-versus-host disease. *Biol Blood Marrow Transplant*. 2002;8:40–46.

5. Vogelsang GB. Advances in the treatment of graft-versus-host disease. *Leukemia*. 2000;14:509–510.

6. Lee SJ, Zahrieh D, Agura E, et al. Effect of up-front daclizumab when combined with steroids for the treatment of acute graft-versus-host disease: Results of a randomized trial. *Blood*. 2004 Sep 1;104(5):1559–1564. Epub 2004 May 11.

13. GRAFT-VERSUS-HOST DISEASE – CHRONIC

In the past, chronic graft-versus-host disease (cGVHD) was characterized by time of onset. Generally speaking, any manifestation of GVHD after day 100 was termed *cGVHD*. The most recent NIH Consensus Working Group data suggests that clinical manifestations, and not the time to symptomatic onset after transplantation, determine if the syndrome is acute or chronic. In addition, a new scoring/grading system replaces the historical system of classifying a patient as having "limited" or "extensive" disease.

There is no consensus to the pathogenesis of cGVHD. T lymphocytes play a major role but evidence shows that in some patients there is coordinated B-cell and T-cell attack. In addition, there is data that suggests that cGVHD may be related to autoimmune reactions of the donor cells.

RISK FACTORS

Accepted Factors

- History of grade II or greater aGVHD
- Disparity at Class I or Class II human leucocyte antigen (HLA) loci
- Peripheral blood stem cells versus bone marrow source
- Patient diagnosis (chronic myelogenous leukemia [CML] and aplastic anemia)
- Female donor → male recipient (even greater if parous)
- Older recipient age
- Multiparous female donor
- History of acute inflammation, for example, TEN, Stevens Johnson, and others
- Non–T-cell-depleted source
- Donor lymphocyte infusion (DLI)
- Sun exposure

Possible Risk Factors

- Cytomegalovirus (CMV) seropositivity
- History of splenectomy

- Corticosteroids as aGVHD prophylaxis
- High number of CD 34^{+} cells in a peripheral blood stem cell infusion

Manifestations

The syndrome of cGVHD may have features that resemble auto-immune and other immunologic disorders such as scleroderma, sjogren syndrome, primary biliary cirrhosis, wasting syndrome, bronchiolitis obliterans, immune cytopenias, and chronic immunodeficiency. The diagnosis is usually clinical and is supported with skin biopsy, Schirmer's test of the eyes, rectal/colonic/oral biopsy, or liver biopsy.

Most cases are diagnosed within the first year and a half following hematopoietic stem cell transplantation (HSCT) but the diagnosis can be as late as several years from transplantation.

Diagnosis of cGVHD

The NIH Working Group recommends that the diagnosis of cGVHD require at least one diagnostic manifestation of cGVHD or at least one distinctive manifestation, with the diagnosis confirmed by pertinent biopsy, laboratory result, or radiology in the same or another organ. A diagnostic sign is one that is explained only by GVHD and therefore, a single sign is sufficient to support the diagnosis. Distinctive signs alone are not sufficient for the diagnosis of cGVHD and therefore require additional testing. It is important that drug reaction, infection, recurrent or new malignancy, and other causes be excluded before diagnosis of cGVHD can be made.[1]

Skin

Diagnostic Manifestations
- Poikiloderma (atrophic and pigmentary changes).
- Lichen planus-like eruptions (erythematous or violaceous-papules or small squamous plaques with or without central lines or silvery or "shining" appearance on direct light).
- Deep sclerotic features (smooth, waxy indurated skin – "thickened or tight skin" callused by deep and diffuse sclerosis over a wide area).

- Morphea-like superficial sclerotic features – (localized patchy areas of smooth or shiny skin, leathery consistency, moveable, often with dyspigmentation).
- Lichen sclerosis-like lesions (discrete to connected gray to white papules of plaques, often with follicular plugs, shiny appearance, leathery consistency and moveable).

Distinctive Manifestations
- Depigmentation, sweat impairment and intolerance to temperature, erythema, maculopapular rash, and pruritis.
- Skin often presents with diffuse mottling and hair may be reduced. In some cases total alopecia beyond the expected time-frame post HSCT may occur.
- Erythema, maculopapular rash, pruritis are commonly seen with both acute and chronic GVHD.

Nails

Distinctive Manifestations
- longitudinal ridging
- nail splitting or brittleness
- onycholysis
- pterygium unguis
- dystrophy
- nail loss

Mouth/Mucous Membranes

Diagnostic Manifestations
- Lichen planus-like changes (white lines and lacy appearing lesions of the buccal mucosa, tongue, palate, or lips.
- Hyperkeratotic plaques (leucoplakia).
- Decreased oral range of motion in patients with sclerotic features of skin.

Distinctive Manifestations
- xerostomia
- mucoceles
- mucosal atrophy
- pseudomembranes
- pain

- ulcers (infectious pathogens such as yeast or herpes simplex virus (HSV) and second malignancies must be excluded)

Features that are common to both acute and chronic GVHD include gingivitis, mucositis, erythema, and pain. Some patients may have gingival hyperplasia from cyclosporine, dilantin, and calcium-channel blockers (especially nifedipine). Patients may benefit from dental consultation with dental service-experienced inpatients undergoing stem cell transplantation.

Sicca syndrome (dry mouth and eyes) is common and is not considered diagnostic because it often reflects gland destruction as an end-stage condition rather than active inflammation.

Eyes

Diagnostic Manifestations
If there is new ocular sicca documented by a low Schirmer test value (both eyes less than or equal to 5 mm) or a new onset of keratoconjunctivitis sicca by slit-lamp examination with mean values of 6 to 10 mm on Schirmer test plus one distinctive manifestation in an other organ, the diagnosis of cGVHD can be inferred, although dry eyes from direct radiation toxicity to lacrimal glands can be confused with cGVHD.

Distinctive Manifestations
- New onset of dry, gritty, painful eyes, cicatricial conjunctivitis, keratoconjunctivitis sicca, and confluent areas of punctate keratopathy.
- Other features include photophobia, periorbital hyperpigmentation, difficulty opening eyes in morning due to mucoid secretions and blepharitis (erythema of the eye lids with edema).
- Severe forms can lead to corneal abrasions.
- Ophthalmology follow-up is also important to assess for cataracts (increased incidence in patients on steroids and/or after TBI).

Genital

Diagnosis of vulvovaginal GVHD relies on symptoms and physical findings. It is reported to occur in about 3% of bone marrow recipients versus 15% of peripheral blood recipients. Most patients with vulvar or vaginal cGVHD have involvement of the mouth or other sites but the vulva or vagina may sometimes be the only site of cGVHD. Mild cases may be asymptomatic and may be detected only on examination.

Diagnostic Manifestations

■   Lichen planus-like features and vaginal scarring or stenosis. The introitus may become narrowed due to scar tissue. Scarring can lead to hair loss and the inability to obtain Papanicolaou smears due to stenosis.

■   Distinctive dryness, fissures, burning, dyspareunia, ulcers (must exclude infection). Patients may benefit from consultation with experienced gynecologist.

Gastrointestinal Tract

Diagnostic Manifestations

Include esophageal web and strictures/stenosis. Features that are common to acute and chronic GVHD include anorexia, nausea, vomiting, diarrhea, weight loss, and failure to thrive. Wasting syndrome may be seen in cGVHD but it is often multifactorial (decreased calorie intake, poor absorption, hypercatabolism). Biopsies should be taken from duodenum, stomach, and esophagus to make the diagnosis. Colonoscopy with biopsy and rectal biopsy should be obtained to assess for lower GI GVHD. Endoscopy findings of mucosal edema and erythema or focal erosions with histological changes of apoptotic epithelial cells and crypt cell dropout may be seen but are not considered diagnostic features. It is important to send stool studies and biopsy samples to rule out infection such as CMV, adenovirus, HSV, Clostridium difficle and so on.

Hepatic acute and chronic GVHD typically present with an increased bilirubin (mostly direct elevation) and increased alkaline phosphatase (usually out of proportion to transaminases). In fewer cases, it can present as acute hepatitis. Liver biopsy shows focal portal inflammation with bile duct obliteration that may progress to sclerosis. The histologies of acute and chronic liver GVHD are similar.

Lung

Bronchiolitis obliterans (BO), is the only diagnostic feature of pulmonary cGVHD. The diagnosis of BO by pulmonary function tests (obstructive disease) and radiologic testing requires at least one other distinctive manifestation in a different organ system to support the diagnosis of cGVHD. Clinical features include dyspnea on exertion (usually in severe cases), shortness of breath, cough, wheeze, and chronic asymptomatic rales. Bronchiolitis obliterans organizing pneumonia (BOOP) is seen in both acute and chronic GVHD.

A working definition of BO from the NIH Consensus is as follows:

1. FEV1/FVC <.7 and FEV1 <75% predicted
2. Evidence of air trapping or small airway thickening of bronchiectasis on chest CT with inspiratory and expiratory cuts, residual volume >120%, or pathologic confirmation of constructive bronchiolitis.
3. Absence of infection in the respiratory tract, documented with investigations directed clinical symptoms, such as radiologic studies or microbiologic cultures.
4. BO – organizing pneumonia not due to infections may represent a manifestiation of either acute or c GVHD and is considered a common feature.

Hematology and Immune System

Cytopenias resulting from stromal damage or autoimmune processes are common in cGVHD but should not be used to establish the diagnosis of cGVHD. Autoantibodies may develop with autoimmune hemolytic anemia and idiopathic thrombocytopenic purpura (ITP). Refractory thrombocytopenia often seen particularly in progressive/continuous onset is associated with the highest nonrelapse mortality (serving as a marker of severity of illness). It is not uncommon to see eosinophilia (>500), lymphopenia (<500), hypogammaglobulinemia, or hypergammaglobulinemia.

Musculoskeletal System

Diagnostics Features
- Fascial involvement associated with sclerosis of overlying tissue, joint stiffness/contractures.
- Fasciitis presents with stiffness, decreased range of motion, edema, dimpling of the skin, and joint contractures.

Distinctive Manifestations
- Clinical myositis with tender muscles and increase in muscle enzymes can occur. Evaluation of myositis involves electromyography and measurement of creatinine phosphokinase

(CK) or aldolase. The diagnosis should be confirmed with muscle biopsy. Arthralgia or arthritis is common.

■ If changes in mobility are noted, early- and long-term involvement with PT/OTis critically important.

Other Manifestations
■ Serositis (pericardial, pleural effusions, or ascites).
■ Peripheral neuropathy.
■ Myasthenia gravis.
■ Nephritic syndrome, and cardiac involvement have been suggested in cGVHD but these manifestations are uncommon.
■ In rare instances, cGVHD is often a diagnosis of exclusion.

Infections

Patients with cGVHD are very susceptible to encapsulated bacteria (due to decreased IgG2, IgG4 synthesis and splenic dysfunction). In patients with cGVHD, opsonization is impaired, and encapsulated organisms (*Neisseria meningitides, Haemophilus influenzae, Streptococcus pneumonia*) may cause rapidly progressive and life-threatening infection. One must remain very alert to this possibility. Continue penicillin and antibacterial prophylaxis, as Bactrim alone may not be enough to prevent pneumococcal disease. (See Chapter 15, bacterial infections.) A common late cause of death is pneumococcal sepsis. *Varicella zoster* occurs frequently in patients with cGVHD.

The risk of late CMV infections is higher in patients with cGVHD. The risk is highest in patients who were treated for early CMV infection.

Other complications to be aware of include sinusitis, recurrent HSV infections, and *Aspergillus* infection. *Aspergillus* infection of the lung or sinuses is the most common late fungal infection in patients on chronic or high dose corticoid steroids to treat cGVHD.

The total immunoglobulin (Ig)G level may be normal but IgG subclasses 2,4 may be low; therefore, fractionate IgG levels. If subclasses are found to be low, consider replacement IV IgG.

SCORING/GRADING

The NIH Consensus Panel developed a new clinical scoring of organ systems grading scale as discussed previously. The new system replaces the current definition that labels patients as having either limited or extensive disease. Use the scoring sheet to score each organ followed by an overall grade of mild, moderate, or severe.

- Mild cGVHD
  - Involves one or two organs or sites with no clinical significant functional impairment.
- Moderate cGVHD
  - At least one organ or site is involved with clinically significant but not major, functional impairment; maximum score of 2 in any affected organ or site, orThree or more organs/sites are involved but with no clinically significant functional impairment; maximum score of 1 in all affected organ/sites, or
  - Chronic GVHD of the lung with a score of 1.
- Severe cGVHD
  - Score of 3 in any organ or site with major disability, or
  - cGVHD of the lung with a lung score of greater than or equal to 2.

Previous grading by defining limited or extensive disease is as follows:

- Limited
  - Characterized by localized skin involvement and/or evidence of hepatic dysfunction.
- Extensive
  - Characterized by either generalized skin involvement or with localized skin involvement or hepatic dysfunction plus at least one of the following:
    - Liver histology showing chronic progressive hepatitis, bridging necrosis or cirrhosis.
    - Involvement of the eye (Schirmer's test with less than 5 mm wetting).
    - Involvement of minor salivary glands or oral mucosa (as demonstrated on labial or mucosal biopsy specimen).
    - Involvement of any other target organ as described in the earlier text on cGVHD.

Organ scoring of chronic GVHD.

	SCORE 0	SCORE 1	SCORE 2	SCORE 3
PERFORMANCE SCORE: ☐	☐ *Asymptomatic and fully active (ECOG 0; KPS or LPS 100%)*	☐ *Symptomatic, fully ambulatory, restricted only in physically strenuous activity (ECOG 1, KPS or LPS 80–90%)*	☐ *Symptomatic ambulatory, capable of self-care, >50% of waking hours out of bed (ECOG 2, KPS or LPS 60–70%)*	☐ *Symptomatic, limited self-care, >50% of waking hours in bed (ECOG 3–4, KPS or LPS <60%)*
KPS ECOG LPS				
SKIN	☐ No Symptoms	☐ <18% BSA with disease signs but **NO** sclerotic features	☐ 19–50% BSA **OR** superficial sclerotic features "not hidebound" (able to pinch)	☐ >50% BSA **OR** deep sclerotic features "hidebound" (unable to pinch) **OR** impaired mobility, ulceration or severe pruritus
Clinical features:				
☐ Maculopapular rash				
☐ Lichen planus-like features				
☐ Papulosquamous lesions or ichthyosis				
☐ Hyperpigmentation				
☐ Hypopigmentation				
☐ Keratosis pilaris				
☐ Erythema				
☐ Erythroderma				
☐ Poikiloderma				
☐ Sclerotic features				
☐ Pruritus				
☐ Hair involvement				
☐ Nail involvement				
% BSA ☐				
Involved ☐				

	No symptoms	Mild	Moderate	Severe
MOUTH	☐ No symptoms	☐ Mild symptoms with disease signs but not limiting oral intake significantly	☑ Moderate symptoms **with** disease signs with partial limitation of oral intake	☑ Severe symptoms with disease signs on examination **with** major limitation of oral intake
EYES Means tear test (mm): ☐ >10 ☐ 6–10 ☐ ≤5 ☐ Not done	☐ No symptoms	☐ Mild dry eye symptoms not affecting ADL (requiring eyedrops ≤3 × per day) **OR** asymptomatic signs of keratoconjunctivitis sicca	☐ Moderate dry eye symptoms partially affecting ADL (requiring drops >3× per day or punctal plugs), **WITHOUT** vision impairment	☐ Severe dry eye symptoms significantly affecting ADL (special eyeware to relieve pain) **OR** unable to work because of ocular symptoms **OR** loss of vision caused by keratoconjunctivitis sicca
GI TRACT	☐ No symptoms	☐ Symptoms such as dysphagia, anorexia, nausea, vomiting, abdominal pain or diarrhea without significant weight loss (5<%)	☐ Symptoms associated with mild to moderate weight loss (5–15%)	☐ Symptoms associated with significant weight loss > 15%, requires nutritional supplement for most calorie needs **OR** esophageal dilation
LIVER	☐ Normal LFT	☐ Elevated Bilirubin, AP*, AST or ALT <2×ULN	☐ Bilirubin >3 mg/dl or Bilirubin enzymes 2–5×ULN	☐ Bilirubin or enzymes >5×ULN
LUNGS† ☐ **FEV1**	☐ No symptoms	☐ Mild symptoms (shortness of breath after climbing one flight of steps	☐ Moderate symptoms (shortness of breath after walking on flat ground)	☐ Severe symptoms (shortness of breath at rest; requiring o2)

(continued)

85

	SCORE 0	SCORE 1	SCORE 2	SCORE 3
PERFORMANCE SCORE: ☐ KPS ECOG LPS	☐ *Asymptomatic and fully active (ECOG 0; KPS or LPS 100%)*	☐ *Symptomatic, fully ambulatory, restricted only in physically strenuous activity (ECOG 1, KPS or LPS 80–90%)*	☐ *Symptomatic ambulatory, capable of self-care, >50% of waking hours out of bed (ECOG 2, KPS or LPS 60–70%)*	☐ *Symptomatic, limited self-care, >50% of waking hours in bed (ECOG 3–4, KPS or LPS <60%)*
DLCO ☐	☐ FEVI > 80% OR LFS = 2	☐ FEVI 60–79% OR LFS 3–5	☐ FEVI 40–59% OR LFS 6–9	☐ FEVI ≤ 39% OR LFS 10–12
JOINTS AND FASCIA	☐ No symptoms	☐ Mild tightness of arms or legs, normal or mild decreased range of motion (ROM) **AND** not affecting ADL	☐ Tightness of arms or legs **OR** joint contractures, erythema thought due to fasciitis, moderate decrease ROM **AND** mild ot moderate limitation of ADL	☐ Contractures **WITH** significant decrease of ROM **AND** significant limitation of ADL (unable to tie shoes, button shirts, dress self etc.)
GENITAL TRACT	☐ No symptoms	☐ Symptomatic with mild signs on exam **AND** no effect on coitus and minimal discomfort with gynecologic exam	☐ Symptomatic with moderate signs on exam **AND** with mild dyspareunia or discomfort with gynecologic exam	☐ Symptomatic **WITH** advanced signs (stricture, labial agglutination or severe ulceration) **AND** severe pain with coitus or inability to insert vaginal speculum

Other indicators, clinical manifestations or complications related to chronic GVHD (check all that apply and assign a score to its severity (0–3) based on its functional impact where applicable (none–0, mild –1, moderate –2, severe –3)

Esophageal stricture or web_____	Pericardial Effusion_____	Pleural Effusions(s)_____
Ascites (serositis)_____	Nephrotic syndrome_____	Peripheral Neuropathy_____
Myasthenia Gravis_____	Cardiomyopathy_____	Eosinophilia > 500 μl_____
Polymyositis_____	Cardiac conduction defects_____	Coronary artery involvement_____
Platelets <100,000/μl_____	Progressive onset_____	

Others: Specify:

---

* Alkaline phosphatase may be elevated in growing children, and not reflective of liver dysfunction.

† Pulmonary scoring should be performed using both the symptom and pulmonary function testing (PFT) scale whenever possible. When discrepancy exists between pulmonary symptom or PFT scores the higher value should be used for final scoring. Scoring using the Lung Function Score (LFS) is preferred, but if DLCO is not available, grading using FEV1 should be used. The LFS is a global assessment of lung function after the diagnosis of bronchiolitis obliterans has already been established. The percent predicted FEV1 and DLCO (adjusted for hematocrit but not alveolar volume) should be converted to a numeric score as follows: >80% = 1; 70% to 79% = 2; 60% to 69% = 3; 50% to 59% = 4; 40% to 49% = 5; <40% = 6. The LFS = FEV1 score + DLCO score, with a possible range of 2 to 12. ADL, activities of daily living; AP, alkaline phosphatase; ALT, alanine aminotransferase; AST, aspartate aminotransferase; BSA, body surface area; DLCO, carbon monoxide diffusing capacity; ECOG, Eastern Cooperative Oncology Group; FEV1, forced expiratory volume; GVHD, graft-versus-host disease; KPS, Karnofsky Performance Status; LFS, Lansky Performance Status; LFTs, liver function tests; LPS, Lansky Performance Status; ULN, upper limit of normal.

THERAPY OF CHRONIC GVHD

Primary

Steroids

Prednisone is the first-line therapy at 1 to 2 mg/kg/day. Consider topical corticosteroids if small area and skin involvement only. If no improvement in symptoms, consider combination of tacrolimus or cyclosporine. Combination therapy can be considered as primary therapy but evidence for this approach is questionable.

Secondary

- Tacrolimus (Prograf, FK-506): Standard oral dosing is 0.05 mg/kg every 12 hours, rounded to the nearest 0.5 mg. Dosing is approximate and levels should be followed per institute standards/protocol. Reasonable target levels are between 5 and 10 ng/mL.
- Cyclosporine: Standard oral dose is 5 mg/kg/dose every 12 hours . Dosing is approximate and levels should be followed per institute standards/protocol. Typical level range is 200 to 400 ng/mL.
- Mycophenolate Mofetil (CellCept, MMF): Standard dose varies. Typical dose is 15 mg/kg orally every 12 hours (1,000 to 1,500 mg/dose) – may need to start low and work dose up slowly, for example, 250 mg every 12 hours → 1,000 mg every 12 hours to manage GI side effects. Advantage is that, it can be given orally or IV. May be added for steroid sparing. This is the most commonly used agent for steroid refractory GVHD.
- Sirolimus (Rapamune): Standard dose is 12 mg load followed by 4 mg/day. Levels should be followed per institute/protocol. Reasonable target levels are between 3 and 12 ng/mL.
- Psoralen Ultraviolet Irradiation (PUVA): Is administered to the skin surface and is used for cutaneous manifestations only. PUVA has been associated with increased risks of skin cancer.
- Extracorporeal photopheresis (ECP): Is when leukocytes are obtained from peripheral blood by apheresis, incubated with

8-MOP, irradiated, and then reinfused to the patient where they undergo apoptosis and induce tolerance.

ECP has been useful in some patients with cGVHD but is used primarily for cutaneous manifestations (especially lichen planus).

- Treatments range per center with 1 to 4 sessions per week.
- Platelets may need to be >50 and hematocrit >30. Helpful to check TIBC, ferritin, and iron levels at the start of therapy since RBC loss during the procedure can result in iron deficiency.

- Thalidomide is selected patients is primarily useful for mucositis and lichen planus. Starting dose is 50 to 200 mg twice daily.

- Rituximab is currently on clinical trial, but does seem to be beneficial in some patients. Response is more favorable in patients with cutaneous and rheumatologic cGVHD. Dose 375 mg/m^2 once a week for 4 weeks. Can treat with a second 4 week course if incomplete response. Important to monitor for known effects of hypogammaglobulinemia.

- Pentostatin (Nipent) is a nucleoside analog that inhibits adenosine deaminase, an enzyme critical for T-cell function. It has some activity in cGVHD but increases susceptibility to infection. It should be used cautiously.

- Topical therapy such as steroids and/or calcineurin inhibitor preparations may be helpful in mild skin GVHD and may allow for lower doses or avoidance of systemic steroid therapy. These medications can be used in combination with one another and with the addition of an antipruritic agent such as pramoxine 1% or hydrocortisone 1%.

Topical Steroids

- Desonide 0.05% applied BID to affected area.
- Triaminolone 0.1% applied BID to affected area.
- Fluocinonide 0.5% applied BID to affected area.
- Clobetasol 0.05% applied BID to affected area. Most potent and is not recommended for use for longer than 2 weeks.
- The aforementioned high dose steroids should not be applied to the face, groin or axilla.

Topical Calcineurin Inhibitors

- Tacrolimus 0.03% or 0.1% applied BID to affcted area.
- Pimecrolimus 1% applied BID to affected area.

SYMPTOM MANAGEMENT AND SUPPORTIVE CARE OF GVHD

Oral cGVHD

Localized and Symptomatic Disease

CORTICOSTEROID GELS

Corticosteroids are directed at specific areas – high potency (fluocinonide) or ultrahigh potency (clobetasol or betamethasone dipropionate).

- Fluocinonide gel 0.05% BID or TID. Comes in 15/30/45/60 g tubes. Dry area thoroughly before applying medication. Avoid food or drink for 30 minutes after use.
- Clobetasol gel 0.05% BID or TID. Comes in 15/30/45/60 g tubes. Dry area thoroughly before applying medication. Avoid food or drink for 30 minutes after use.
- Betamethasone dipropionate gel 0.05% BID or TID. Comes in 15/30/45/60 g tubes. Dry area thoroughly before applying medication. Avoid food or drink for 30 minutes after use.

High-potency steroids should not be applied to the vermillion border of the lip because they will cause irreversible atrophy.

Alternative to corticosteroids is tacrolimus ointment (Protopic). Protopic is a vaseline-based ointment which is generally less effective in the mouth than alcohol-based corticosteroid gels. It is a good option for the treatment of "chapped lips" caused by GVHD.

- Tacrolimus ointment (0.1%) BID or TID. Comes in 30/60/100 g tubes. Areas should be thoroughly dried before ointment is applied. Avoid food or drink for 30 minutes after use.

Corticosteroid rinses directed at entire oral cavity. Dexamethasone is the most commonly used rinse. Patients should be counseled for the potential of oral thrush and need for anticandidal therapy. Patients who have significant ulcers and inflammation may have more systemic effects of topical therapy with the ultrapotent steroids.

- Dexamethasone 0.5 mg/5 mL. Swish 5 to 10 mL (encourage the patient to swish for 4 to 6 minutes if possible) and then spit 4 to 6 times/day. Food and drink should be avoided for 30 minutes after use.
- Prednisolone 15 mg/5 mL. Swish 5 to 10 mL (encourage patient to swish for 4 to 6 minutes if possible) and then spit

4 to 6 times/day. Food and drink should be avoided for 30 minutes after use.

- Triamcinolone 0.1% aqueous solution. Swish 5 to 10 mL (encourage patient to swish for 4 to 6 minutes if possible) and then spit 4 to 6 times/day. Food and drink should be avoided for 30 minutes after use.Triamcinolone intralesional injections every 3 to 4 weeks may be helpful in patients who fail to respond to topical therapy.

Xerostomia (Salivary Gland cGVHD)

Patients with dry mouth have variable oral sensitivities to hot, cold, spicy and acidic food, mint (toothpaste), and carbonated beverages. Patients may also develop mucoceles (blisters on the palate and inside of the lower lip). Symptomatic mucoceles must be distinguished from herpetic lesions. Mucoceles may respond to topical steroids or topical analgesics. Deep mucoceles require surgical excision especially when symptomatic.

Interventions for xerostomia include frequent water sipping, mouthwash without alcohol, artificial saliva products, children's toothpaste (may be less irritating), ultrasoft tooth brush, sour sugarless candies, biotene mouth wash. It is important that patients are getting adequate fluoride in an attempt to prevent dental caries. Flouride treatments should be performed before bed without rinsing. Patients without subjective oral dryness should use additional fluoride to prevent tooth decay.

- Analgesia can substantially alleviate symptoms of dry mouth and can be helpful when symptoms impair nutrition or communication. Examples include viscous lidocaine, 2% solution 5 mL, swish and spit PRN or Maalox-Benadryl-Lidocaine (1:1:1) 5 mL, swish and spit PRN.
- Cholinergic agonists may also be helpful if they result in a significant enhancement of salivary gland secretion and can be offered in the absence of contraindications such as glaucoma, heart disease, or asthma. We have found that some patients have experienced improvement using pilocarpine (Salagen) 5 mg PO BID or cevimeline (Evoxac) 30 mg TID.
- If possible, avoid xerogenic medications such as tricyclic antidepressants, selective serotonin reuptake inhibitors (SSRI)s, antihistamines, and narcotics.

Gastrointestinal cGVHD

Odynophagia

Confirming the diagnosis is very important. Sometimes endoscopy is needed to exclude or to confirm. Other causes of odynophagia or dysphagia can include pill esophagitis, esophageal webs/rings/strictures, esophageal dysmotility or radiation esophagitis, and fibrosis. Lubrication and esophageal dilation may be helpful in patients with documented strictures.

Diarrhea cGVHD

Patients must have a standard work-up including screening for infectious causes, malabsorption, lactose intolerance, gall bladder disease, medication induced. Workup may include endoscopy and biopsy.

Obtaining an accurate history may help with diagnosis. A history may indicate that the diarrhea is malodorous, suggesting malabsorption, or the diet may indicate lactose intolerance, which is common after transplantation. Pancreatic enzyme supplementation is helpful in patients with diarrhea and malabsorption.

Medications such as MMF or magnesium supplementation may cause diarrhea. Magnesium with protein (mineral bound to soy protein) may help eliminate the laxative effects.

If there is no clear etiology, referral to a gastroenterologist experienced in transplant patients is strongly recommended. Nutritional support is important, as more than 40% of patients with cGVHD are malnourished. Some patients will require total parenteral nutrition or tube feedings.

Hepatic cGVHD

The use of ursodeoxycholic acid (Actigall) 300 mg TID can be used as an adjunct to help reduce liver injury and perhaps improve pruritus in some patients.

Ocular cGVHD

Dry eyes is a common complaint, and lubrication should be offered to all patients. Preservative-free lubricating artificial tears will coat the ocular surface, minimizing superficial punctuate keratopathy reducing ocular symptoms and improve vision.

- Patients may tolerate certain formulations better than others. Encourage them to try different brands. Common brands include Refresh, Refresh Plus, Refresh PM (ointment), Systane, Bion, TheraTears, celluvisc, Tears Naturale, Lacrilube ointment, and Hypotear ointment.

- For patients who require artificial tears more than once every hour, lacriserts may be helpful. They are slow-dissolving 5 mg pellets of hydroxypropyl methylcellulose (prescription only). The lacrisert is inserted daily into the inferior cul-de-sac of the eye. Patients may not tolerate the insert because it can have a foreign body sensation. Oral medications can be used in an attempt to stimulate tear flow.

- All patients should be encouraged to perform warm compress and do routine lid care to maximize the output of the meibomien glands (the outer oil layer of the tear film).

- Flax seed oil (2 tablespoons of oil twice daily – capsules are not recommended) can create a healthier oil-tear layer but must be used with caution in patients with liver dysfunction.

- Doxycycline 20 mg BID or 50 mg daily has been used to treat rosacea blepharitis by reducing inflammation on the lids (avoid if issues with photosensitivity).

- Refractory cases should be referred to a specialist with experience in treating cGVHD. Boston Scleral Lens Prosthetic Device are large contact lenses that trap a thin layer of saline next to the cornea. They are often helpful with very severe dry eyes. They are not generally available but inquiries can go to www.**bostonsight**.org.

- For patients in whom drainage is a problem, temporary silicon plugs or permanent occlusion (cauterization) can be used.

- The use of topical steroid may be necessary, especially in the setting of a flare of GVHD while tapering systemic steroids but should be used under the care of an ophthalmologist.

- Clofazimine 300 mg/day for 90 days, and then dropping the dose to 50 mg/day may be of some value for scleroderma.

Genital cGVHD

Patients with cGVHD of the genitalia should be followed closely by a gynecologist with experience in treating cGVHD.

General hygiene

- Avoiding mechanical and chemical irritants.
- Clean genital area with warm water rather than soap or feminine products.
- Area should be dried thoroughly with air or counsel patient to dry front to back.
- Emollients such as pure vitamin E oil can be applied very sparingly to help retain natural moisture. Emollients should only be applied to external genital area, not internally.
- Lanolin cream (small amounts) can be used to relive itch and irritation, provided there is no abnormal discharge present.
- Replens or other bacteriostatic gels may be used in the vagina to alleviate dryness. Replens adheres to the vaginal wall and is intended to last longer than water-soluble gels typically used as sexual lubricants.
- Low estrogen states – If vulvovaginal cGVHD is accompanied by low estradiol levels, topical estrogen therapy with or without the use of a vaginal dilator should be initiated unless contraindicated (increased risk of breast cancer or cardiovascular events etc.).
- Local treatment of vulvovaginal cGVHD – If the only clinical manifestation of cGVHD activity is local and mild, topical immunosuppressive therapy may constitute an adequate primary therapy. If there is other clinical activity, systemic therapy plus topical is likely necessary. Systemic immunosuppressive therapy is indicated for vulvovaginal GVHD that is refractory to topical measures or progresses or develops during treatment.
- Sclerotic features of the vagina should be treated aggressively. Application of high-potency corticosteroid is the mainstay of therapy, although the use of topical calcineurin ointments has been reported.
- Betamethasone dipropionate augmented gel or ointment 0.05% (15/50 g tube). Apply topically to the vulva and/or 1 gm intravaginally (using vaginal estrogen cream calibrated applicator) every 12 to 24 hours for upto 12 weeks.
- Tacrolimus 0.03% and 0.1% ointment – apply a thin layer to affected areas twice daily (store at room temperature).
- It is important that infections such as *Human papiloma* virus (HPV), HSV, *Candida*, bacteria, or other recognized

gynecologic pathogens be excluded before and periodically during the use of topical therapy. Gynecologic evaluations should be performed at regular intervals during treatment, sooner if new or worsening symptoms occur.

- Surgical lysis with or without vaginal reconstruction is necessary for extensive synechiae and complete obliteration of the vaginal canal.

Pulmonary cGVHD

Recent studies indicate that pulmonary function (PF) decline during the first year post transplantation is significantly associated with a higher mortality risk. Early changes in PF tests detected 100 days after transplant do not reflect changes that may occur later in the transplant course.

Complications such as airflow obstruction, bronchiolitis obliterans (BO), and bronchiolitis obliterans with organizing pneumonia (BOOP) are most likely to occur between day 100 and 1 year, during which time immunosuppression is weaned. See section on pulmonary complications for more details.

Gastroesophageal reflux (GERD) and silent aspiration must be considered in cGVHD patients with airflow limitation in the setting of postnasal drip and/or recurrent sinus infections occur.

Treatment
- Systemic steroids.
- Prophylactic IVIG in the setting of recurrent sinus infections.
- Inhaled corticosteroids and bronchodilators.
- Pulmonary rehabilitation programs.
- Supplemental oxygen (if SpO_2 <87% while breathing room air). The amount of oxygen should be titrated using a 6-minute walk conducted according to the American Thoracic Society Guidelines.
- Possibly ECP.
- Early referral for early consideration of lung transplantation is appropriate for certain candidates. Interventions pioneered in lung transplantation and cystic fibrosis management such as inhaled cyclosporine, amphotericin or tobramycin, and rotating empiric antibiotics have not been rigorously tested in the cGVHD setting.

Hematopoetic Effects of cGVHD

Cytopenias are often seen in the setting of cGVHD.

■ Thrombocytopenia: At the time of diagnosis of cGVHD, thrombocytopenia is associated with a poor prognosis. It may be due to ITP and thus be responsive to IVIG or rituximab treatment.

■ Eosinophilia: Eosinophilia is seen in both acute and chronic GVHD. It is associated with elevated levels of IL-5 and can herald or represent disease activity.

NEUROLOGIC COMPLICATIONS OF cGVHD

Chronic GVHD can result in neurological complications such as polyneuropathy, myositis, and myasthenia. These symptoms may manifest as muscle weakness, wasting, pain, burning, dysethesias, and paresthesias. Central nervous symptoms such as cerebral angiitis and vasculitis/encephalitis are less clearly associated with cGVHD.

A complete physical and neurological examination is required to investigate neurological symptoms in people with cGVHD. The care and treatment of patients with cGVHD with neurological findings primarily rests on ruling out other etiologies for neuropathic changes. Things to consider include calcineurin inhibitors, proximal muscle steroid myopathy, inflammatory myopathy, chronic inflammatory demyelinating polyneuropathy, polymyositis, myasthenia gravis, and nerve root compression fracture.

FOLLOW-UP

Careful multiorgan system follow-up and medication review is required monthly. Important labs to monitor include specific drug levels, complete blood count (CBC), complete panel including renal and liver function, and IgG levels. Careful attention should be paid to iron studies, lipid profile, and endocrine function and PFTs as needed. Involvement of occupational therapy/physical therapy, ophthalmology, dental, dermatology, and other subspecialties as needed such as gynecology and neurology as indicated. Infections pose serious risk. All patients should be formally evaluated in setting of fever. Protective precautions should be extended in this population beyond 6 to 12 months. Mortality is high, often due to infection, in extensive cGVHD.

INFECTION PROPHYLAXIS

General guidelines include monthly IVIG to maintain IgG levels >400. (Seattle group reported decreased nonrelapse mortality above this level.) PCN/Amoxicillin or macrolide for prophylaxis against encapsulated organisms, Bactrim or continued other PCP prophylaxis for duration of immunosuppressive therapy. Penicillin prophylaxis may be recommended to decrease risk of infection from *Streptococcus pneumoniae*, which is seen in spite of Bactrim prophylaxis. Many centers recommend continued infection prophylaxis with Bactrim/penicillin and monthly IVIG until 6 months after cessation of immunosuppression. However, increasing resistance of *Pneumococcus* to PCN makes this strategy questionable.

Prophylaxis against PCP, *Varicella zoster,* and HSV should continue in patients with or being treated for cGVHD.

REFERENCE

1. Filipovich AH, Weisdorf D, Pavletic S, et al. National Institutes of Health consensus disease I. Diagnosis and staging working group report. *Biol Blood marrow Transplant.* 2005;11(12):945–956.

14. ENGRAFTMENT SYNDROME

Engraftment syndrome is an inflammatory disorder that usually occurs within the first 2 weeks after stem cell transplantation.

CLINICAL MANIFESTATIONS

Clinical manifestations may be associated with high fevers, generalized erythrodermatous rash, and third-spacing (explaining peripheral and noncardiogenic pulmonary edema). There may be cough, dyspnea, hypoxemia, multilobar pulmonary infiltrates, or other nonspecific findings.

DIAGNOSIS

Diagnosis is one of exclusion. There is no test for it, but tests that may be undertaken to rule out alternative etiologies include cultures, skin biopsy, and bronchoalveolar lavage.

ETIOLOGY

Etiology is poorly understood. In general, it is thought to reflect cytokine production due to immune dysregulation in the context of neutrophil recovery. The polymorphonuclear leukocytes (PMN) and lymphocytes are thought to be activated and contribute to the injury through further production of inflammatory mediators.

DIFFERENTIAL DIAGNOSIS

- Hyperacute graft-versus-host disease (GVHD) or traditional GVHD.
- Infection: Patients should always be treated presumptively for infection while diagnostic studies and cultures are being carried out.
- Transfusion-associated lung injury (TRALI). This entity typically occurs proximate to a transfusion and is thought to be due to preformed antiHLA antibodies in the transfused product.
- Drug reaction.

TREATMENT

Modest dose corticosteroids – for example, 40 mg solumedrol IVB daily followed by a taper if there is a response. No standard exists, but engraftment syndrome is generally very responsive to doses of steroids often considered too low to be effective in acute GVHD. If there is a prompt response, the steroids can be tapered rapidly over 10 to 14 days.

15. INFECTIOUS DISEASE

Risk factors for infection include the degree and duration of neutropenia; profound pan-immunosupression; disruption of mucosal barrier by radiochemotherapy; HLA mismatch; central venous access; and donor infectious states. Inadequate immunoglobulin (Ig) G2 and IgG4 production increases risk of infection with encapsulated organisms despite total Ig levels in the normal range post transplant.

Please see Chapter 18 for specific pulmonary infections.

GENERAL TIME FRAMES OF WHEN INFECTION IS LIKELY TO OCCUR

- Day 0 to 30: Infections related to conditioning regimen and neutropenia (bacteremias of gastrointestinal or catheter-related origin), invasive aspergillosis related to neutropenia, candidemia.
- Day 30 to 80: Classic opportunistic infections (*Cytomegalovirus* [CMV], *Pneumocystis jiroveci* pneumonia [PCP], toxoplasmosis, nocardiosis, invasive aspergillosis, and other invasive mold infections related to severe GVHD).
- Day 180+: Encapsulated organisms (especially in patients with chronic GVHD [cGVHD]), *Varicella zoster* virus [VZV], PCP. Risk for viral and fungal infections protracted in unrelated donor HSCT.

Figure 15.1 outlines the period of the major host deficits and infections that occur during allogeneic HSCT in relation to when targeted pathogen-specific prophylactic, preemptive, and empiric therapies are deployed. Risk for infectious complications is temporally dependent and significantly decreased in the setting of prophylactic, preemptive, or empiric therapy. The risk of certain infections after transplantation is highly associated with ongoing immunologic manipulation as seen with the therapy for GVHD (linkages noted by vertical arrows).

Standard prophylactic considerations in this context include GNR – trimethoprim/sulfamethoxazole (TMP-SMX) or fluoroquinolone; Candida species – fluconazole; PCP – TMP-SMX, atovaquone, dapsone, or pentamidine; and HSV/VZV – acyclovir.

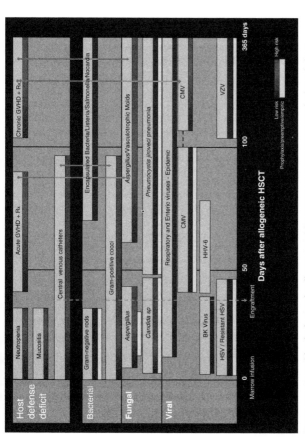

Figure 15.1 Timetable of infection for allogeneic HSCT patients receiving antimicrobial prophylaxis.

CVL, central venous line; GVHD, graft-versus-host disease; GNR, gram-negative rods; GPC, gram-positive cocci; PCP, *Pneumocystis jiroveci* pneumoniae; CMV, *Cytomegalovirus*; HHV-6, *Human herpes virus-6*; HSV, *Herpes simplex virus*; VZV, *Varicella zoster virus*.

Standard emipiric therapeutic considerations in this setting include GNR – ceftazidime, piperacillin/gentamicin, or imipenem; *Aspergillus*/molds/*Candida* – amphotericin preparations or extended spectrum azoles; and CMV – IV ganciclovir, valganciclovir, or preemptive monitoring (by antigenemia or polymerase chain reaction [PCR]).

FEVERS

The response to fevers depends on the clinical situation. For nonneutropenic patients who become febrile during conditioning, we usually pan-culture but do not start antibiotics unless the patient looks ill or is rapidly becoming neutropenic. Temperatures during neutropenia demand cultures and broad-spectrum antibiotics targeting gram-negative organisms. Options for first-line therapy for febrile neutropenia include third- or fourth-generation cephalosporin +/− vancomycin. In general, use of vancomycin is not recommended but may be appropriate for selected patients if the patient is known to be colonized with *Staphylococcus aureus* from surveillance cultures or if there is significant skin breakdown, concerns about indwelling catheter sites, or positive results of blood cultures for gram-positive bacteria before final organism identification/sensitivities or if the patient is unstable with hypotension or other signs of sepsis.

For patients allergic to cephalosporins, piperacillin and aminoglycoside can be used. Cefepime can also be used because the cross-sensitivity with ceftazidime is <1%. Avoid aztreonam because it shares the same side chain as ceftazidime and there is possible cross-reactivity between these two agents; anti-*Pseudomonas* activity of aztreonam is not optimal.

Third-line fever and neutropenia therapy includes imipenem, piperacillin-tazobactam, or aztreonam plus levofloxacin. It is important to consider your hospital algorithms and resistance to organisms.

Empirical antifungal therapy is often reserved for persistent fevers >96 hours after starting empiric antimicrobials targeting gram-negative bacteria. However, patients with long periods of neutropenia or those on steroids may be at higher risk for fungal infection.

We also suggest baseline and once or twice weekly labs for serum galactomannan (*Aspergillus* antigen) assay and/or serum 1-3-β-Glucan assay.

Patients receiving piperacillin-tazobactam may have false positive galactomannan assays. Patients who have recently received intravenous gammaglobulin (IVIG) or albumin may have false positive glucan tests.

Isolated Fevers

All patients who are receiving immunosuppressive drugs for GVHD should be evaluated emergently for fever >101°F regardless of time from transplantation. Patients should be instructed to monitor their temperature at home. Patients who are not receiving immunosuppressive drugs should be evaluated on an individual basis.

In general, the greater the disparity between donor and recipient, the poorer the functional reconstitution of the immune system (despite normalization of their counts). Therefore, isolated fevers of >101°F should be evaluated on the basis of the nature of the donor and the presence of GVHD and its treatment. Autologous and related allogeneic transplant patients without GVHD/medications should be seen within the first 6 months of transplantation, and allogeneic patients (especially with unrelated donors) should be seen in the emergency room (ER) within the first 9 to 12 months (longer if on immune suppression). These are guidelines; if clinical suspicion or unusual presentation appears, patients should be evaluated.

Patients on steroids may be seriously ill with temperatures 100°F to 100.5°F and should be seen emergently with aggressive empiric therapy.

Any patient with central access needs to have cultures drawn from the periphery and from the line. Central lines should be removed promptly for most bacteremias other than *Staphylococcus epidermidis.*

BACTERIAL INFECTION

Infection rates are lower with prophylactic oral antibiotics during transplantation. Late post-HSCT infections are associated with immune suppression and GVHD. Some data suggest a decrease in infection rates in patients given prophylactic immunoglobulin.

Some confusion has arisen as to the indications for penicillin prophylaxis in patients post-HSCT. There is minimal literature on this topic. The only well-substantiated indication appears to be for patients who have active chronic GVHD and are thus at risk for encapsulated organism infections who cannot tolerate (TMP-SMX). In addition, some patients (generally those with cGVHD) have markedly decreased splenic function after HSCT marked by Howell–Jolly bodies on their smear. Such patients are appropriate candidates for routine penicillin prophylaxis. Daily SMX-TMP provides pneumococcal prophylaxis. Certain strains of *S. pneumoniae* are resistant to TMP-SMZ and penicillin, and if these are given thrice weekly, it will not prevent pneumococcal disease. For patients who are unable to take TMP-SMZ and pneumococcal prophylaxis as desired, amoxicillin 500 mg PO BID is recommended.

Gammaglobulin

Intravenous gammaglobulin (IVIG) should not be administered routinely for bacterial infection prophylaxis. Patients with severe hypogammaglobulinemia should receive replacement. Patients should be monitored routinely (every 4–12 weeks). The goal should be to maintain serum concentrations above 400 to 500 mg/dL. Frequency and dose can be adjusted as needed but a useful starting point is 500 mg/kg once per month.

Allogeneic HSCT recipients with normal IgG levels may have low IgG2 and IgG4 subclasses with normal total IgG levels. Since IgG2 and IgG4 subclasses are important in clearing encapsulated organisms, low subclass levels may be associated with a high risk of sepsis despite otherwise normal-appearing IgG levels. IVIG may be useful in treating some severe viral infections.

VIRAL INFECTION

Cytomegalovirus *(CMV)*, HSV, VZV, Adenovirus, Epstein-Barr virus (EBV), and Human herpes virus-6 (HHV-6) are common non-respiratory viral complications in transplantation. Influenza and respiratory viruses such as parainfluenza type III and Respiratory syncytial virus (RSV) are also common serious concerns.

Cytomegalovirus

Cytomegalovirus is more common in the allogeneic transplant population and usually occurs between 2 and 6 months post-HSCT. All HSCT candidates and allogeneic donors should be screened for evidence of CMV immunity. The highest-risk patients are those who are CMV seropositive and receive cells from a CMV seronegative donor and those receiving T-cell-depleted or cord grafts. Posttransplant acute GVHD increased the risk of CMV reactivation and disease.

All HSCT patients should receive leukocyte-reduced or CMV-seronegative red blood cells (RBCs) and platelets to prevent transfusion-associated infection.

Prophylaxis

The Infectious Diseases Society of America (ISDA) recommends that all HSCT patients at risk should begin one of two CMV disease-prevention programs at the time of engraftment to continue through day 100 or later if the patient is still on immunosuppressive agents.

The first strategy is to administer prophylactic ganciclovir/valganciclovir through day +100. The second strategy is to take preemptive action against early CMV infection. This involves routine weekly screening for evidence of CMV reactivation. Treatment is started if the screening test becomes positive. The screening method requires highly sensitive and specific laboratory tests so that rapid initiation of therapy can be done. Diagnostic methods used for screening may include antigenemia testing or other DNA-based assay. In highly immunocompromised patients, it is reasonable to screen weekly for a longer period of time, but there is no consensus on frequency of duration.

It is recommended that centers without access to routine CMV testing should use the prophylatic approach, recognizing that ganciclovir is myelosuppressive and that there may be an increased risk of bacterial infections.

There continues to be a small risk (<5%) of transfusion-related acquisition of new CMV infection; thus CMV monitoring is appropriate in CMV-negative donor and recipient .

Preemptive therapy is administered for a high or rising CMV viral load. Oral valganciclovir is the current preferred antiviral agent for preemptive therapy of CMV viremia. Alternative treatments include the use of IV ganciclovir or foscarnet.

Treatment

Valganciclovir 900 mg every 12 hours daily for induction until virus clears, followed by 900 mg daily for another 2 to 4 weeks.

Recipient CMV status	Donor CMV status	Reactivation (%)
+	+	60–70
+	–	60–70
–	–	0–5
–	+	10–20

CMV DISEASE (COLITIS, PNEUMONITIS, GI)

■ Ganciclovir 5 mg/kg IV every 12 hours ×10 to 14 days or oral valganciclovir (900 mg orally every 12 hours) until symptoms and signs of the disease resolve and viremia clears, followed by suppressive doses (900 mg/day) for an additional 2 to 4 weeks.

■ Foscarnet 60 mg/kg IV over 1 hour every 8 hours for 2 to 3 weeks (induction dose) depending on clinical response plus IVIG 500 mg/kg Monday, Wednesday, and Friday for six doses. The dose of 90 mg/kg IV over 1.5 to 2 hours every 12 hours can be used but we find that there is an increased level of nephrotoxicity at this dose and hence routinely use the 60 mg/kg IV dosing regimen. Check calcium, magnesium, and potassium levels at least twice daily until replacement requirements are established. Foscarnet should always be initiated in the hospital.

■ Ganciclovir 5 mg/kg every 12 hours for 10 to 14 days + IVIG 500 mg/kg thrice weekly for six doses.

■ Leflunomide 100 mg/day loading dose followed by 20 to 50 mg daily in conjunction with ganciclovir, valganciclovir, or foscarnet may be useful in patients with resistant disease.

■ Newer agents such as maribivir may soon be available.

■ CMV-IG or IVIG may be useful in CMV pneumonia. The suggested dose is 500 mg/kg every other day for six doses. Its value in other forms of CMV disease is uncertain.

Herpes Simplex Virus

Infections can be almost 100% prevented with the use of antiviral prophylaxis.

Prophylaxis

Universal prophylaxis should be instituted in all patients beginning with conditioning regimen and continuing until a year posttransplant or longer if systemic immunosuppression is continued beyond a year. It is reasonable to continue prophylaxis for 2 months after all systemic immunosuppression is discontinued. HSV-seronegative patients should be educated on the importance of avoiding direct contact with any potentially infected person.

- Acyclovir 400 mg PO TID, 800 mg PO BID, or 200 mg IV TID, adjusted for decreased renal function.
- Valacyclovir 500 mg orally twice daily or 1,000 mg once daily, adjusted for decreased renal function.

Treatment

- Herpetic mouth sores
  - Confirm infection with culture. If the culture is negative, consider empiric therapy and biopsy by oral medicine or otorhinolaryngology service.
- Lips only
  - Acyclovir 400 mg PO 5 times/day.
  - Famciclovir 250 mg PO TID.
  - Valacyclovir 1,000 mg PO BID.
- Oral ulcers
  - Severe mucositis, cutaneous disease.
  - Acyclovir 250 mg/m^2 or 5 mg/kg every 8 hours (IV dose adjusted for renal function). PO conversion is based on weight and renal function. Treat for 4 weeks if cGVHD is present. Some patients may require IV therapy for resistant infections.

Varicella Zoster

Prophylaxis

Reactivation as shingles is common late after HSCT with an incidence of approximately 50% to 60%. VZV can disseminate. Family members, household contacts, and health-care workers should be vaccinated if not naturally immune. All HSCT recipients should avoid exposure to persons with active VZV infection. Acyclovir, famciclovir, and valacyclovir prophylaxis is effective but can delay presentation until after the prophylaxis has been discontinued. Varicella zoster occurs frequently in patients with cGVHD. VZV hyperimmunoglobulin should be administered to patients 96 hours after close contact with a person with varicella or shingles if still immunocompromised. If VZV hyperimmunoglobulin is not available, we recommend using treatment doses of valacyclovir or famciclovir beginning on day 5 of the exposure for 14 days. If the patient experiences a varicella zoster virus–like rash after contact with or exposure to a person with varicella or herpes zoster, antiviral therapy should be administered.

- Acyclovir 400 mg PO TID or 800 mg PO BID, adjusted for decreased renal function.
- Valacyclovir 500 mg orally daily, adjusted for decreased renal function.

Treatment
- Famcyclovir 500 mg PO TID.
- Valacyclovir 1,000 mg PO TID.

VZV-seronegative
Immunocompromised HSCT recipients who are exposed to varicella should be treated with acyclovir and VZIG as soon as possible but ideally within 96 hours of the exposure or with treatment doses of valacyclovir/famcyclovir as mentioned earlier.

Treatment
- Acyclovir 10 mg/kg IV TID for disseminated VZV (>1 dermatome involved or evidence of pulmonary or hepatic involvement).
- Valacyclovir 1,000 mg TID or famiciclovir 500 mg PO every 8 hours can be used for limited disease.

Severe abdominal pain that mimics acute cholecyctitis or appendicitis should be considered visceral VZV and treated empirically until proven otherwise. This occurs in approximately 10% of post-HSCT zoster.[1,2]

Epstein–Barr Virus

Another serious herpes virus complication of immunosuppression is the development of Epstein-Barr virus–related lymphoproliferative disorders (EBV-LPD). In contrast to most lymphomas, EBV-LPD tends to occur in extranodal sites, such as the brain and gastrointestinal tract. Depending on the degree of immunosuppression administered, it has been reported in up to 25% of patients with organ transplants and a similar number of patients with stem cell grafts. Typically, it occurs in recipients of T-cell-depleted or cord grafts and is uncommon in standard transplantation using calcineurin inhibitors and methotrexate. This presumably relates to some degree of passive immunity transmitted with the donor T cells. These tumors often can be detected when they represent a polyclonal proliferation of EBV-transformed B cells. Local radiotherapy, systemic chemotherapy, and the administration of humanized monoclonal antibodies directed against B cells (rituximab) are sometimes useful. Administration of T cells from the donor intravenously may reestablish effective immunity. Such an approach can be quite effective but runs the risk of inducing GVHD. Systematic monitoring of EBV viral load should be considered in these subpopulations.

Human Herpes Virus-6

Reactivation has been associated with pancytopenia, pneumonitis, and encephalitis. It can be established by assessing the viral load by PCR, although many patients after HSCT will have low viral loads that appear to be innocuous. Making the diagnosis is important since the virus usually responds to foscarnet therapy. In general, the risk of reactivation is higher in more immunocompromised patients, for example, after T-cell depletion or cord-blood transplantation.

Adenovirus

Morbidity varies from mild respiratory illnesss to fulminant disseminated infection with hepatic failure and high mortality. The latter scenario is rare.

No specific antiviral treatment is of proven efficacy for these infections. Cidofovir seems to be active in vitro and has been used on some occasions, but the data are anecdotal at this time.

Treatment

Cidofovir – 5 mg/kg intravenously every week for the first 2 weeks. This is followed by a minimum of four doses every other week.

Prehydrate aggressively before each dose and administer with probenecid.

Respiratory Syncytial Virus

These viruses can cause significant morbidity/mortality; the spectrum of infection ranges from mild upper respiratory illness to viral pneumonitis. Secondary bacterial or fungal infections do occur, especially early after transplantation. Strict contact precautions and use of mask and gloves in the inpatient and outpatient areas continue to be the best strategy in preventing these infections. Transplantation should be delayed if Respiratory syncytial virus (RSV) is diagnosed around the expected transplant date. Reference Chapter 18 for more information .

Treatment
There is no proven treatment. Seek and aggressively treat secondary infections. Ribavirin aerosolized 6 g daily over 18 hours has been used in the past, but is no longer thought to be useful in RSV pneumonia although some institutions continue to use it.

IVIG 500 mg/kg QOD for 5 to 7 days may be helpful.

Influenza

All HSCT patients should be treated independently of the duration of symptoms. Providers should be vigilant for secondary bacterial or fungal infections that may occur following or concomitant with influenza. Vaccination of all household members is recommended with killed vaccine preparations before the beginning of the influenza season. All recipients should be vaccinated yearly following HSCT.

Treatment
- Zanamivir 10 mg inhaled BID.
- Oseltamivir 75 mg PO BID – for influenza A or B. Adjust for renal dysfunction.
- Amantadine 100 mg BID ×10 days or rimantadine 100 mg PO BID – for influenza A only.

Pneumocystis Jiroveci Pneumonia

Prophylaxis

Hematologic malignancy patients are at a much higher risk of developing PCP than solid tumor patients. PCP can develop early after transplantation, especially in patients who were heavily treated before the HSCT. Risk may extend beyond a year, particularly if immune suppressive medications are continued or reinstituted.

It is recommended that prophylaxis be initiated no later than 30 days post-HSCT and continued for at least 1 year or longer if the patient remains on immunosuppressant therapy for GVHD. PCP rarely occurs before day +50 after HSCT, unless corticosteroids are used before or during transplantation.

Trimethoprim/sulfamethoxazole (TMP-SMX) 80/400 mg daily is the most effective agent. Once platelet count is 50 to 100 K or higher and ANC >1,000, TMP-SMX is preferred. Alternatives include 160/800 mg thrice weekly. Leucovorin (folic acid) 25 mg by mouth weekly may help prevent associated myelosuppression if it occurs.

Daily TMP-SMX provides significant prophylaxis against other opportunistic pathogens such as *Nocardia*, *Toxoplasma gondii*, *Isospora belli*, *Cyclospora cayetanensis*, susceptible strains, or *S. pneumoniae*, *Haemophilus influenzae*, and common gram-negative GI and GU bacteria.

- Atovaquone 750 mg PO BID or 1,500 mg PO daily if unable to take TMP-SMX.
- Dapsone 50 mg by mouth twice daily. Most common toxicities include rash, hemolytic anemia, and methemoglobinemia. It can not be given to patients with glucose-6-phospate dehydrogenase (G6PD) deficiency and should not be given to allogeneic recipients of G6PD-deficient donors. Note that even people without G6PD deficiency may hemolyze.
- Pentamidine IV (loading dose) 4 mg/kg × 3 doses either daily or thrice weekly. Then 4 mg/kg every 2 weeks. Nephrotoxicity, hepatotoxicity, and hypoglycemia can occur.
- Aerosolized penatmidine 300 mg monthly. May not provide adequate coverage because of poor distribution throughout the lung and therefore is not encouraged. Adverse reactions include bronchospasm. In the absence of contraindications, when ordering aerosolized penamidine we recommend a PRN order for bronchodilators.

Treatment:

- TMP-SMX (high dose) with adjuvant glucocorticoids. TMP-SMX 15 to 20 mg/kg/day (IV or orally) divided every 6 to 8 hours. Prednisone (begin as early as possible and within 72 hours of PCP therapy) 40 mg PO BID days 1 to 5, 40 mg orally QD days 6 to 10, then 20 mg orally QD days 11 to 21.
- Atovaquone 750 mg PO TID.
- Dapsone/primaquine – dapsone 100 mg PO daily + primaquine 15 mg PO daily.

FUNGAL INFECTION

Invasive fungal infections are an important cause of death in HSCT patients. The most common fungal infection in HSCT is candidiasis, but Aspergillus occurs in 5% to 15% of patients and the risk is associated with local environmental factors, duration of neutropenia, and corticosteroid use. Prophylaxis is recommended in the allogeneic patient population and in autologous patients who have underlying hematologic malignancies or are very heavily pretreated and whose local risk of invasive disease is greater than 15%.

Two serum tests, β-glucan and galactomannan may be valuable adjuncts when making the diagnosis. Galactomannan is specific for all species of *Aspergillus* and *Penicillium*. β-Glucan will test positive for all fungal infections with the exception of cryptococcosis and zygomycosis. False-positive galactomannan results may occur if the patient is receiving piperacillin, piperacillin-tazobactam or Plasma-lyte. False-positive β-glucan results may occur if the patient is receiving IVIG, cefazolin, IV augmentin (reports in Europe), gauze in serosal surfaces (abdominal or chest packing), or cellulose-containing dialysis membranes.

Prophylaxis

- Nystatin swish and swallow – 5 mL PO TID.
- Fluconazole 200 to 400 mg PO daily.
- Voriconazole 6 mg/kg IV every 12 hours as loading dose and then 4 mg/kg IV every 12 hours followed by 200 mg orally every 12 hours. The role of voriconazole in prophylaxis has not been determined..
- Posaconazole 200 mg orally TID.

Monitor cyclosporine, tacrolimus, sirolimus levels and LFTs when the patient is on an azole drug since they may increase immuno-suppressant levels and LFTs.

Treatment

Candida species

- Echinocandins
  - Caspofungin (cancidas) 70 mg IV daily one followed by 50 mg IV daily.
  - Micafungin (mycamine) 100 mg IV daily.
  - Anidulafungin 200 mg load dose on day 1, followed by 100 mg daily.
- Azoles
  - Fluconazole if sensitive species – 800 mg load, followed by 200 to 400 mg orally daily.
  - Voriconazole – initial, 6 mg/kg IV every 12 hour for 2 doses, then 3 mg/kg IV every 12 hour; may switch to oral dosing as tolerated.
  - Posaconaozle (Noxafil) 400 mg every 12 hours for refractory oropharyngeal candidiasis, not approved for candidemia; 200 mg TID is the prophylaxis regimen. Should be taken with a meal or oral supplement.
  - Itraconazole (Sporanox) – 200 mg (oral, capsules or solution) every 12 hours. IV therapy 200 mg IV every 12 hours × 2 days and continues with 200 mg orally every 12 hours.
- Amphotericin B liposomal (AmBisome) – 3 to 5 mg/kg/day IV once daily, infused over at least 120 minutes.

Aspergillus

- Azoles
  - Voriconazole (preferred agent) – initial, 6 mg/kg IV every 12 hours for 2 doses, then 4 mg/kg IV every 12 hours; may switch to oral dosing as tolerated. Maintenance, 200 to 300 mg orally every 12 hours for patients weighing over 40 kg; 100 to 150 mg orally every 12 hours for patients under 40 kg.
  - Posaconazole – 200 mg orally QID or 400 mg orally BID, only if refractory to amphotericin B or voriconazole (no data on use as first-line agent at this time).

- Itraconazole
  - ORAL, 200 mg to 400 mg daily.
  - IV, 200 mg infused over 1 hour twice daily for four doses, then 200 mg once daily.
  - Life-threatening situations, ORAL, 200 mg three times daily for 3 days, then ORAL 200 mg daily; treatment should continue for at least 3 months.
  - Life-threatening situations, IV, 200 mg twice daily for four doses, then IV 200 mg daily; continue for at least 3 months.
- Echinocandins
  - For patients who are refractory or intolerant to voriconazole or amphotericin only. There is no good data to support use as first-line agent.
  - Caspofungin 70 mg IV day one followed by 50 mg IV daily.
  - Micafungin 150 mg IV daily (possibly higher doses, but not an approved indication).
- Amphotericin B liposomal (AmBisome) – 3 to 5 mg/kg/day IV once daily, infused over 120 minutes.

Zygomycosis

- Amphotericin B liposomal (preferred agent) – 5 mg/kg/day IV once daily, infused over 120 minutes. Daily dosing could be increased to 7.5 to 10 mg/kg, depending on severity.
- Azoles
  - Posaconazole – 800 mg/day orally divided BID to QID (for salvage or step-down treatment. No data on primary efficacy to date).

HEPATITIS B AND C

It is important to identify donors with previous history or chronic infection with hepatitis B or C to decide if the donor is suitable. It is also important to identify, evaluate, and manage recipients with previous or chronic infection with hepatitis B or C to minimize impact of these infections during transplantation.

Hepatitis C – Donor

Treatment in the donor is important in preventing long-term complications as well as in dealing with HCV transmission.

Donors who are found to be HCV-IgG positive should have liver function tests performed, and a quantitative HCV RNA evaluation if not already done.

Donors who are HCV-IgG positive with negative HCV RNA should be informed of the abnormality and may donate stem cells. The recipient in this case would be monitored to assess the HCV viral load serially (every 2 months) for the first 6 months after transplantation. If the patient becomes HCV-RNA positive that patient will then be considered for treatment following engraftment after consultation with infectious diseases and hepatology service.

Donors who are HCV-IgG and HCV-RNA positive should be triaged according to the donor's health status, availability of alternate donors, and patient's disease. If there is no risk to the donor and the disease necessitates prompt transplantation, the donor could still be considered suitable (refer to your institution's Standard Operating Procedure [SOP] regarding recipient consenting requirements) and the recipient would be informed about the risks and benefits of proceeding in this situation. After the stem cells are collected, the donor can be referred for therapy and if there is time the donor should be offered antiviral therapy with the goal of eliminating circulating HCV RNA. If the donor is considered unsuitable, an appropriate alternative donor should be sought. All donors who are HCV-RNA positive are considered ineligible and institutional SOP should address consenting ineligible donors and their recipients in appropriate situations (Figure 15.2).

Hepatitis C – Patient

For patient with unknown HCV status, current screening involves measurement of anti-HCV IgG and quantitative HCV RNA. Patients who are known to be infected with HCV, or are identified through screening process, should undergo a quantitative HCV RNA measurement, HCV genotyping, and a liver biopsy if these procedures have not been done within a year of the HSCT procedure, independent of LFT results.

Assessment should include risk of the transplant if cirrhosis is present, risk of progression to cirrhosis, and overall HCV-related survival depending on biopsy results, other comorbiditites, and the prognosis of the primary hematologic malignancy.

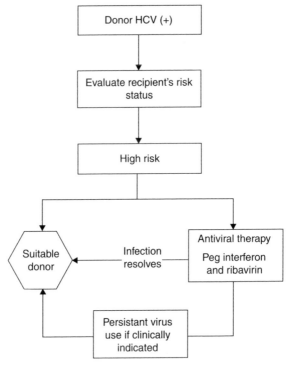

Figure 15.2 Hepatitis C infected donor flow chart.

HCV, *Hepatitis C* virus.

If there is no cirrhosis and the patient has low-risk disease, transplantation can be performed after a trial of appropriate antiviral therapy if deemed appropriate.

Hepatitis B – Donor

Donors should be routinely screened by testing for HBV surface antigen (HBsAg) and HBV core antibody (HBcAg). If both tests are negative, donors can proceed. Donors, who screen positive for either test, should undergo further testing for detection of HBV surface antibody (HBsAb) and measurement of a quantitative HBV virus load if possible. Donors who are

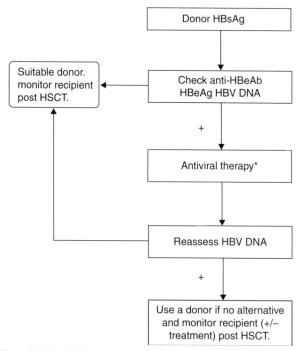

Figure 15.3 Hepatitis B infected donor flow chart.

* Current treatment include lamuvidine, adefovir, entecavir.

HBeAg, Hepatitis B virus e antigen; HBsAg, Hepatitis B virus surface antigen.

HBsAb positive and HBV-virus-load negative can donate without problem (previous, resolved infection). Donors who are HBsAg positive or HBV-virus-load positive should be referred to an infectious disease or hepatology service for further evaluation and management as soon as possible to decide on donor appropriateness, donor treatment strategies, and timing of donation. Patients with aggressive diseases and no alternative donor, a donor with HBV DNA or HBeAg can be used if there is no alternative donor with an appropriate posttransplant antiviral strategy designed in consultation with ID and/or hepatology service (Figure 15.3).

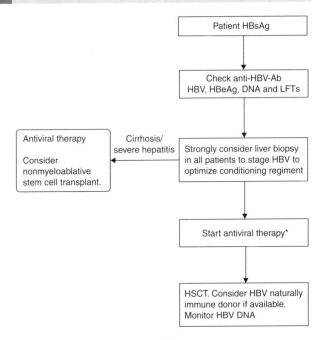

Figure 15.4 Hepatitis B recipient patient flow chart.

* Current treatment include Lamuvidine, Adefovir, Entecavir (referral to ID or GI strongly recommended).

HBV, *Hepatitis B* virus; HBV-Ab, Hepatitis B virus antibody; HBeAg, Hepatitis B virus e antigen; HBsAg, Hepatitis B virus surface antigen; LFT, liver function test.

Hepatitis B – Recipient

Recipients are currently screened by testing for HBsAg and HBcAb. Initial testing for HBsAb should be considered. If all tests are negative, transplant can proceed without problem. HBV vaccination is contemplated for all recipients post transplant.

If the patient is HBsAb positive and HBcAb negative (previously vaccinated), transplant can be done. Recipients who screen positive for HBsAg or HBcAb positive should undergo further testing for detection of HBV surface antibody (HBsAb) and measurement of a quantitative HBV virus load. All patients with positive HBsAg or detectable HBV virus load should be evaluated.

The evaluation should include measurements of HBsAg, HBeAb, HBeAb HBV genotyping, and a strong consideration for liver biopsy for appropriate staging before transplant.

Patients who are HBcAb positive, but with no evidence of chronic HBV infection, should be monitored posttransplant by measurements of HBV virus load every 2 months for the first year after transplant. An HBV-immune donor should be selected if available. If HBV virus load is detected post-HSCT, these patients should be referred to an infectious disease or hepatology service for further evaluation and management. If patients develop chronic GVHD and need ongoing systemic immunosuppression or if patients develop abnormal LFTs after transplantation, rescreening with HBsAg and/or HBV virus load should be considered periodically, even after the first year after HSCT. Infectious disease or hepatology consultants will often dictate the timing and nature of HBV antiviral treatment. As this field is rapidly evolving, no specific antiviral treatment is discussed here (Figure 15.4).

REFERENCES

1. Locksley RM, Flournoy N, Sullivan KM, Meyers JD. Infection with varicella-zoster virus after marrow transplantation. *J Infect Dis.* 1985 Dec;152(6):1172–1181.

2. Han CS, Miller W, Haake R, Weisdorf D. Varicella zoster infection after bone marrow transplantation: Incidence, risk factors and complications. *Bone Marrow Transplant.* 1994 Mar;13(3):277–283.Infectious Disease

16. GRAFT REJECTION AND FAILURE

GRAFT REJECTION

- Graft rejection refers to the immunologic rejection of donor hematopoietic elements by the residual host immune system. Graft rejection occurs more frequently in patients transplanted for aplastic anemia and in patients receiving unrelated or mismatched transplants (because of increased donor–recipient disparity at major and minor HLA loci). Graft rejection may also be observed in reduced-intensity regimens, especially in patients who are not pretreated heavily.

- In many patients with aplastic anemia, the underlying pathophysiology reflects an autoimmune recognition of the stem cells by an aberrant immune response. Most conditioning regimens used in aplastic anemia are reduced-intensity regimens. If the conditioning regimen does not fully eliminate the abnormal immune response, the graft may fail by the same mechanism that resulted in aplastic anemia in the first place. Prior to matched related donor transplantation, family member, directed donor transfusions should not be administered to avoid alloimmunization of the patient against minor histocompatibility antigens that are common to other family members.

GRAFT FAILURE

- Graft rejection must be differentiated from the non–immune-mediated graft failure associated with inadequate stem cell numbers or stem cell viability or possibly a microenvironment defect with the stem cell niche (also termed graft exhaustion). The latter can be inferred when there is full donor chimerism but no hematologic recovery. Myelotoxic medications may be implicated as well. Often, drugs such as, sulfamethoxazole-trimethoprim, valganciclovir, mycophenolate mofetil, and others are used concomitantly and may have additive myelosuppressive activity. Ironically, the precise infections and conditions treated with these myelosuppressive agents may also suppress hematopoiesis. *Cytomegalovirus* (CMV), human herpes virus type 6 (HHV-6),

Varicellazoster virus (VZV) and other infections may cause depression of counts that may be slow to recover. Infection should always be considered when assessing the cause of graft failure. It may be difficult to distinguish rejection from other causes of graft failure, but chimerism analysis is the most useful test to differentiate these phenomena.

- In umbilical-cord blood transplantation, both graft rejection and stem cell failure may be the concerns. Most cord-blood transplantation is performed across HLA barriers, providing a strong potential stimulus for graft rejection. Moreover, the viability of a cord blood product cannot be assessed until after the unit is thawed. Sometimes these units have suboptimal CD34$^+$ cell counts, suggesting either preservation of a unit with a low stem cell number, or loss of cells during cryopreservation.

- Preexistent HLA antibodies are an important risk factor for graft rejection. Multiparous women or patients who are heavily transfused may make antibodies against HLA antigens. It is important to check the serum for these antibodies prior to selecting a mismatched stem cell product of any kind. Once graft rejection occurs, it is useful to look for these antibodies again to allow selection of a donor with a different HLA type.

TREATMENT

- Treatment of graft failure is by infusion of another stem cell product. There are no definitive data to determine the best stem cell product for infusion; however, if full chimerism is detected we recommend a CD34-selected (or T-cell depleted) product to avoid the additional risk of GVHD.

- Treatment of graft rejection also requires administration of another stem cell product. It is likely that in patients with graft rejection, chimerism analysis will show few if any donor cells. In this setting it is likely that additional conditioning will be required. There are no commonly accepted regimens that are used in this context. However, typically it is desirable for the regimen to be highly immunosuppressive without adding a lot of organ toxicity. Such regimens often include alemtuzumab, fludarabine, and/or antithymocyte globulin as well as other cytotoxic agents or low dose TBI. T-cell depletion (or CD34 selection) should be avoided. In fact, if the transplanted product was bone marrow, often a peripheral blood stem cell transplant is used to provide a large number of T cells that may suppress the antistem cell immune response. As noted above, if the original graft was mismatched and there are HLA antibodies present, it is important to try and choose a donor whose HLA-type is not reactive with those antibodies.

■ The mortality after graft failure is high, primarily due to the increased risk of opportunistic infections related to the extended duration of neutropenia.

17. GASTROINTESTINAL COMPLICATIONS

NAUSEA/VOMITING

Chemotherapy and/or radiation are typically emetogenic, and symptoms are expected early after hematopoietic stem cell transplantation. Medications such as antibiotics, opioids, MMF, mepron, and others can also contribute to nausea and vomiting. Acute upper gastrointestinal (GI) graft-versus-host disease (GVHD) typically manifests as nausea and can only be reliably diagnosed by biopsying the stomach. Infections with Herpes simplex virus (HSV), cytomegalovirus (CMV), adenovirus, *Heliobacter pylori*, and fungus are common offenders and need to be treated specifically.

Pattern

- Acute onset occurs within 24 hours of chemotherapy administration (peak at 4 to 6 hours) and lasts for 24 to 48 hours. Usually responds to drug therapy.
- Delayed onset occurs more than 24 hours after chemotherapy administration (peak at 2 to 3 days) and can last for several days. Variable response to drug therapy – commonly seen with cyclophosphamide, anthracyclines, and cisplatin.
- Delayed after engraftment, usually associated with weight loss; may be GVHD.

Diagnostic Testing

- Upper endoscopy with biopsy may be useful to assess for either GVHD or infectious etiologies.

Management

It is preferable to prevent as much nausea and vomiting as possible since treated established nausea is more difficult to manage. Moreover, prevention will decrease future anticipatory, breakthrough and delayed nausea/vomiting.

Anticipatory nausea/vomiting may best be controlled with anti-anxiety medications and behavioral interventions. Delayed nausea should be treated with scheduled antiemetics for 2 to 4 days after the completion of chemotherapy. Antiemetics used in combination provide greater protection than antiemetics used alone. Do not use two antiemetics from the same class as it will significantly increase risk of side effects.

- Serotonin antagonists – 5HT-3 antagonists: ondansetron (Zofran), palonsetron (Aloxi), granisetron (Kytril), dolansetron (Anzemet). Standard therapy for highly emetogenic regimens in combination with steroids. Also has efficacy in XRT mediated nausea/vomiting. Side effects include headache, elevated liver function tests (LFTs), diarrhea or constipation, dizziness, hyperkalemia (palonsetron). May cause QTc prolongation, especially in combination with other QT-prolonging agents. Palonsetron has a very long half-life (several days) and should not be used concomitantly with ondansetron or granisetron, although it may be used repeatedly at the time of chemotherapy administration.

- Steroids – dexamethasone: These are not commonly used in allogeneic HSCT. If necessary, they should be used for a short duration.

- Substance P/neurokinin 1 (NK1) receptor antagonists: Aprepitant/Emend. This drug can be used in conjunction with a 5HT-3 antagonist with dexamethasone. Aprepitant may interact with tacrolimus, rapamycin, and cyclosporine as well as with chemotherapy agents and must be used with caution in these patients. It is primarily metabolized by CYP3A4 in the liver.

- Phenothiazines: Compazine, Trilafon. Useful for nausea/vomiting associated with various etiologies. Flexible routes of administration.
  - Mechanism of action is as antidopaminergics.
  - Side effects: Sedation, hypotension, extrapyramidal side effects (EPS). EPS reactions are characterized by prolonged tonic contractions. They occur with rapid onset or are delayed up to 96 hours after the last dose or dose increase. Presentation may include akathisia, trismus, glossospasm, tongue protrusion, pharyngeal-laryngeal dystonia, blepharospasm, oculogyric crisis, torticollis, and retrocollis.
  - Treatment includes either Benadryl 50 mg or Cogentin 2 mg. Relief is typically seen within 5 minutes; may repeat in 15 minutes if no response. Ativan may be more effective for akathisia.

- Butyrophenones: Haldol, Droperidol (Inapsine). Effective dose in cancer patients is 2.5 to 5 mg IV every 3 to 4 hours. Works as antidopaminergic. Toxicity is similar to phenothiazines but with less sedative effects. Concern about QTc prolongation requires the use of monitoring.
- Benzodiazepines: Lorazepam (Ativan). This drug is best used in combination with other antiemetics; not truly an antiemetic but has amnestic, anxiolytic, and sedative properties. Its side effects include sedation, hypotension, disinhibition and hallucinations, motor incoordination.
- Zyprexa (Zydis – sublingual): This is a useful agent that is used in low doses, seems to be an effective breakthrough agent. Side effects include tachycardia, extrapyramidal reactions, sedation, and glucose intolerance.

Preventive Regimens

- Ondansetron (Zofran) 8 mg IV every 8 hours or 24/ 32 mg IV daily. Administer on days of chemotherapy + additional 24 to 48 hours (for delayed effects). Some patients benefit with slightly longer administration.
- Granisetron (Kyrtil) 1 mg IV every 12 hours. Administer on days of chemotherapy + additional 24 to 48 hours (for delayed effects). Some patients benefit with slightly longer administration.
- Palonosetron (Aloxi) 0.25 mg IV. Dose during transplantation has not been established. It has a very long half-life so it may be adminstered QOD or Q 3 days *plus* prochlorperazine (Compazine) 5 to 10 mg PO or IV before chemotherapy, then every 6 hours PRN +/– diphenhydramine 25 mg *plus* lorazepam (Ativan) 1 to 2 mg IV before chemotherapy and every 6 hours PRN or another serotonin antagonist plus dexamethasone 2 to 10 mg IV or orally can be used with any of the above treatment regimens. Use for a short duration of time and if possible, avoid in the allogeneic stem cell transplant setting.

Breakthrough Nausea/Vomiting

- Change prochlorperazine to 10 mg IV every 6 hours and add diphenhydramine 25 to 50 mg IV every 6 hours PRN EPS reaction.

- If patient tolerates oral agents, change prochlorperazine to 15 mg spansules every 8 to 12 hours.
- If ineffective, stop prochlorperazine and consider adding haloperidol 1 to 2 mg IV every 4 hours +/− diphenhydramine or Zyprexa (Zydis) 2.5 mg to 5 mg orally every 12 hours.
- If ineffective, start metoclopramide (Reglan) 0.5 to 2 mg/kg IV every 6 hours. Its side effects are similar to phenothiazines – diarrhea. It is common to give concurrent benadryl or cogentin with this dose. It is highly effective for chemotherapy-induced nausea/vomiting.
- Dronabinol (Marinol) should be considered if the above regimen continues to be ineffective. Start with 5 mg every 8 hours and increase to every 6 hours (max dose is 10 mg). It has a slow onset of action (days), but also increases appetite.
- Nausea/vomiting associated with motion such as sitting up or moving can be ameliorated with the use of either scopolamine patch 1.5 mg patch every 72 hours or hydroxyzine 25 mg orally every 4 hours.

Delayed Nausea/Vomiting

- Aprepitant (Emend) 125 mg orally on day 1 of chemotherapy, 80 mg orally on day 2 and 3. To be given with decadron 4 to 12 mg orally with each dose.

DIARRHEA

Diarrhea is a common problem both during the HSCT and afterward. The etiology can vary from chemotherapy and/or radiation, GVHD, infection, antibiotics or other drugs, opioid withdrawal, bacterial overgrowth, and lactose intolerance. Multiple etiologies such as GVHD and infection may coexist. CMV, adenovirus, *Clostridium difficile* or extended spectrum beta-lactamase organisms (ESBL) are important etiologies that must be assessed regularly.

Timing

- During conditioning up until day +15 to 20 when mucosal regeneration is typically completed; chemotherapy/radiation and medication are the most common causes of diarrhea.

■ Diarrhea that persists or begins after day +21 should be evaluated for GVHD and infection.
■ Opioid withdrawal can also result in a few days of watery diarrhea as the patient is being readied for discharge.

Diagnostic Testing

■ Stool studies for bacterial, viral, and parasitic agents (if indicated).
■ Endoscopy with biopsy to assess for GVHD and infection. Of note, CMV viral load can be negative in serum but the biopsy can be positive in the intestinal tract, indicating local disease. CT can be helpful in showing bowel wall thickness but it cannot differentiate between GVHD and infection. Severe abdominal pain and/or peritoneal signs may be signs of severe infection, perforation, and GVHD and require immediate intervention.

Management

■ General measures
  - Treat infection, if present, with appropriate antibiotics.
  - Discontinue medications that can contribute to diarrhea. It is important to avoid antidiarrheals until *C. difficile* infection has been ruled out.
  - Assessment of the patient's diet should be considered and if necessary the patient should be started on liquids or made NPO until diagnosis is confirmed and symptoms improved. See GVHD diet recommendations.
  - Lactose intolerance is common after HSCT and low-lactose diet is often useful. It is important to ensure adequate hydration, monitor electrolytes, and continually assess for infection.
  - If GVHD is suspected (high suspicion in all allogeneic patients peri and post engraftment) endoscopy with biopsy (see GVHD section) is required.
■ Noninfectious diarrhea/chemotherapy-/XRT-related
  ▪ Loperamide hydrochloride (Imodium) 4 mg orally followed by 2 mg after each loose stool, upto 24 mg daily.
  ▪ Diphenoxylate hydrochloride/atropine sulphate (Lomotil) 2 tablets or 10 mL solution orally QID until control is

achieved. Decrease to amount needed to maintain control. Maximum daily dose is 20 mg. The atropine will exacerbate dry mouth. Deodorized tincture of opium 0.6 mL orally every 4 to 6 hours either PRN or scheduled. If uncontrolled or patient is unable to tolerate oral intake, octreotide (Sandostatin) – upto 300 µg/hr.

MUCOSITIS

Mucositis and its associated pain and infection risk are one of the principal morbidities of HSCT. Mucositis is caused by injury to the epithelium from conditioning regimens and/or methotrexate. It may involve the entire aerodigestive tract. It is worse in patients who have had prior local radiotherapy in the head and neck region. The injury is probably exacerbated by oral flora penetrating the damaged mucosa. Severe mucositis can lead to severe pain, hemorrhage, infection, upper airway edema, and airway compromise. In the most severe cases endotracheal intubation may be required. Close attention to dental hygiene before transplant is critical. The risk of severe mucositis may be reduced by oral decontamination or palifermin (Kepivance). Kepivance must be administered before the initiation of conditioning therapy and for several days after initiation of conditioning. It has been shown to reduce the severity and duration of mucositis in a total body irradiation (TBI)-based autologous setting, although these protective effects are expected to extend to the allogeneic setting as well. The most common side effects include rash, oral dysesthesia, tongue discoloration, and tongue thickening, and alteration of taste may occur within a week of commencement.

Supportive care includes opioids, oral hygiene, and debridement. All irritants should be avoided. TPN may be required. It should be noted that other common conditions can have similar appearance to oral mucositis. They include fungal infection, HSV, and GVHD.

Dry Mouth

Dry mouth is due to either conditioning regimen injury to salivary glands, anticholinergic agents, or chronic GVHD. Often the cause is multifactorial.

Treatment

- Try to increase oral moisture using fluids or sugar-free candy.
- Civemeline or pilocarpine may be helpful. Dry mouth substantially increases the risk of caries, so fluoride therapy with agents such as Prevident is very important.

INFECTION

Varicella zoster virus reactivation can result not only in well-known cutaneous manifestations, but also (especially in severely immunocompromised patients) in severe abdominal pain without dermatomal vesicles. It is critical to suspect this entity early and treat it aggressively, because it has a significant propensity to dissemination (Chapter 15).

18. PULMONARY COMPLICATIONS

Pulmonary injury is one of the most common complications of stem cell transplantation and a major cause of morbidity and mortality. Damage to the lungs can be multifactorial, including infection, chemotherapy toxicity, graft-versus-host disease, radiation injury, hemorrhage, and immune reactions. Potential etiology can be determined by carefully considering timing of pulmonary complications and if the radiographic studies are focal or diffuse. Important to consider is history including exposures to infectious agents, current and recent prophylaxis regimen, cytomegalovirus status of patient and donor, prior treatment and exposure to pulmonary/cardiotoxic therapy and current and recent immunosuppression thearpy.

All patients should have baseline pulmonary function tests (PFTs) before transplantation, and aggressive diagnostic approach should be taken early after transplantation if there are pulmonary problems.

In general, patients with dyspnea and normal chest X-ray (CXR) should undergo PFTs and arterial blood gas analysis. Restrictive physiology should prompt a chest CT to look for interstitial disease. In patients who have normal PFTs and CXR, cardiac causes such as pulmonary hypertension and cardiac dysfunction should be excluded.

Bronchoscopy with bronchoalveolar lavage (BAL) should be performed early in the search for a diagnosis. If no diagnosis is made, lung biopsy if possible should be considered. Patients with focal infiltrates should be given empiric antibiotics plus or minus fungal therapy and assessed for a response before invasive measures are taken.

INFECTION

Infections are the most common causes of lung injury after transplantation. It is important to consider the entire treatment course including interval post transplant (early or late), medications the patient is on, and the type of transplantation the patient received to come up with a reasonable differential diagnosis for infection. Not only do we need to be concerned about the usual causes of in-hospital and community-acquired pneumonia, but there should also be a general recognition that a variety of unexpected organisms can cause pneumonia. After day +30, bronchoalveolar lavage (BAL) is recommended in an attempt to isolate and treat the organism.

Bacterial Infections

These most commonly occur in the first month but can occur anytime. Both gram-negative and gram-positive organisms can cause pneumonia. Most common organisms include *Escherichia coli, Klebsiella, Pseudomonas, Enterobacter, Acinetobacter, Staphylococcus aureus,* coagulase-negative *Staphylococcus, Streptococcus pneumonia, Streptococcus viridans, Enterococcus.* One also needs to recognize the risk of mycoplasma and chlamydia infections, although the common use of fluoroquinolones will empirically treat these organisms. Other causes of late pneumonia that should not be missed include *Nocardia, Listeria, Actinomyces.*

Viral Causes of Pneumonia

These include CMV, *Herpes simplex* virus (HSV), *Varicella zoster* virus (VZV), adenovirus, *Respiratory syncytial* virus (RSV), influenza, *Parainfluenza* type III, *Herpes virus-6* (HHV-6), metapneumovirus, and a variety of other respiratory pathogens. Non-CMV viral infections may occur earlier than 30 days or later in the transplant course. CMV typically occurs after 30 days. Early detection of CMV and advances in treatment have reduced disease and mortality associated with CMV disease. VZV can lead to pneumonia with or without classic vesicular rash. HSV/VZV prophylaxis should be initiated with the conditioning regimen and continue for 1 year or until they are off all immunosuppressant agents and have recovered CD4 numbers. Community-acquired viral infections can be lethal, especially parainfluenza type III. Since with the exception of influenza there is no effective therapy, the best approach is prevention through isolation.

Diagnosis
Diagnosis is based on fever, cough, signs/symptoms URI, nasal washing, viral swabs, or PCR.

Fungal Pneumonia

Causes of fungal pneumonia include *Aspergillus, Candida, Fusarium, Mucor* and other vasculotrophic moulds. *Candida* and *Aspergillus* are the most common. There is concern about increasing incidence of *Rhizopus* as well as other less common moulds. Refer to Chapter 15 for prophylaxis with fluconazole or voriconazole or posaconazole, and concern about use of steroids predisposing to fungal infections. Monitoring via β-glucan and galactomannan may be helpful.

Diagnosis
- Fever, pleuritic chest discomfort, dyspnea
- Imaging shows nodules or cavitary infiltrates
- The classic "halo sign" may be seen on chest CT but imaging may not be impressive. BAL may be useful.

PNEUMOCYSTIS JIROVECI PNEUMONIA
Risk of *Pneumocystis jiroveci* pneumonia (PCP) starts around day + 30. Effectively taken prophylaxis eliminates PCP.

Diagnosis
- Fever, cough, +/− hypoxemia
- Positive BAL. CXR – bilateral ground glass infiltrates
- A history of noncompliance with prophylaxis medication should be elicited. Typically involves the brain, heart, and lung. Biopsy established by Giemsa stain.

Mycobacteria

Testing with PPD is often not helpful after allogeneic stem cell transplantation because of depressed delayed-type hypersensitivity reactions. Therefore a skin reaction with PPD will likely not occur.

Diagnosis
Culture sputum sample/BAL *M. haemophilum*. Diagnosis should be considered in patients who have skin nodules or joint inflammation with or without pulmonary infiltrates. Diagnosis requires special microbiology culture conditions.

IDIOPATHIC PNEUMONIA SYNDROME

This entity refers to noninfectious pneumonias with several clinical presentations. These complications typically occur around the time of engraftment or neutrophil recovery and again 3 to 6 months post transplantation. Idiopathic pneumonia syndrome (IPS) is more common after allogeneic stem cell transplantation. By definition, there is no identifiable infectious source.

Risk Factors
Allogeneic transplantation – IPS is rare in autologous HSCT, although it can occasionally be related to high-dose cyclophosphamide or other chemotherapeutic agents such as the addition of busulfan. Prior mediastinal radiation increases the risk in patients treated with total body irradiation (TBI). GVHD per se is not well associated with idiopathic pneumonia in humans; however, the risk is increased in patients receiving MTX for GVHD prophylaxis.

Diagnosis
- Cough, dyspnea, crackles, hypoxemia, restrictive physiology,
- Increased alveolar–arterial oxygen gradient, multilobar pulmonary infiltrates, or nonspecific findings on CXR or CT.
- BAL cultures must be negative for infection.
- Lung biopsy shows primarily mononuclear infiltrate into septae; peribronchial and perivascular cuffing present. Typically it occurs within the first 21 days after SCT, although late forms certainly can be observed.

Etiology
These processes are poorly understood. In general, it is thought to reflect conditioning-related lung injury on a background of immunologic injury. Clearly, there may also be undiagnosed infections from common viral infections such as CMV as well as uncommon organisms for example, metapneumovirus.

Differential Diagnosis
The first concern is always to exclude an infection. Patients should always be treated presumptively for a variety of infections while diagnostic studies and cultures are being carried out. A second possible etiology is transfusion-associated lung injury (TRALI). This entity typically occurs proximate to a transfusion and is

thought to be due to preformed anti-human leukocyte antigen (HLA) antibodies in the transfused product. Other causes such as volume overload, cardiac dysfunction, and renal failure must be excluded.

Treatment
High-dose steroids: 1 to 2 mg/kg/daily for 3 days and taper by 50% every 3 days; if given early, may be efficacious. Clinical trials are currently underway to evaluate newer agents such as tumor necrosis factor (TNF) blockers – entanercept (Enbrel).

DIFFUSE ALVEOLAR HEMORRHAGE

This is an acute form of noninfectious respiratory failure occurring within the first month of SCT. It is characterized by progressively bloodier BAL fluid. Ultimately there is diffuse alveolar damage. Mortality is high.

Risk factors
Similar as for IPS mentioned earlier.

Diagnosis
- Progressive cough, dyspnea, crackles, hypoxemia, multilobar pulmonary infiltrates, or nonspecific findings
- BAL fluid is bloody and fails to clear with lavage
- Lung biopsy shows diffuse alveolar damage
- CXR shows diffuse interstitial and alveolar infiltrates that are usually bilateral. Typically, it occurs within the first 21 days after SCT although late forms certainly can be observed.

Etiology
A common thread appears to be disordered cytokine production by engrafting cells – especially TNF. TNF-α infusions in animals result in a DAH-like picture. Moreover, there are provocative data that TNF-α inhibitors such as etanercept (Enbrel) may reverse the process in some patients.

Differential Diagnosis
The first concern is always infection, especially angioinvasive fungi such as *Aspergillus*. Patients should always be treated presumptively for a variety of infections while diagnostic studies and

cultures are being carried out. Serologic tests such as galactomannan assay and β-glucan can be helpful if positive.

Treatment

Data regarding the use of corticosteroids are limited. Given that there may be an infectious component and a baseline immune defect, the use of steroids should be carefully considered. High-dose steroids 1 to 2 mg/kg daily for 3 days and tapered by 50% every 3 days, if given early, may be efficacious. Clinical trials are currently underway to evaluate newer agents such as TNF blockers such as entanercept (Enbrel).

The use of recombinant Factor VII in refractory cases may be considered but the risks of thrombotic events must be carefully considered.

BRONCHIOLITIS OBLITERANS

Bronchiolitis obliterans is the narrowing of small airways leading to air trapping. There is an association with chronic graft-versus-host disease (GVHD) and may be aggravated by infection. This typically is also associated with hypogammaglobulinemia and may be triggered by an infectious pneumonia. It occurs beyond 3 months from transplantation.

Diagnosis

- Dry cough, dyspnea, and wheezes more than crackles
- CXR may show hyperinflation and flattening of diaphragm or may be normal
- Chest CT is the best radiographic study to see narrowing of small airways

Pulmonary function tests show obstructive pattern; reduced spirometry with normal diffusing capacity for carbon monoxide (DLCO). A reasonable set of guidelines has been suggested by the Blood and Marrow Transplantation Clinical Trials Network.

Pulmonary function tests

- Significant obstructive change – decrease of FEV1 by ≥10%, in comparison to pretransplant values, with an FEV1/FVC < 0.7.
- Significant air-trapping – residual volume ≥120%.

NIH proposed definition

- FEV1 <75% of predicted and FEV/FVC < 0.7.
- Clinically – dry cough, dyspnea, and wheezing. No fevers. Signs of chronic GVHD (cGVHD).

Radiology

- CXR – normal or hyperinflation.
- Chest CT – hypoattenuation, bronchial dilatation, bronchiecatsis, presence of centrilobar nodules, and/or expiratory air trapping.
- BAL – nonspecific

Other

- Absence of infection, documented with investigations directed by clinical symptoms, such as radiological studies (radiographs or CT) or microbiologic cultures (sinus aspiration, upper respiratory tract viral screen, sputum culture, or BAL).
- Transbronchial lung biopsy is not diagnostic.
- Open or video-assisted thoracoscopic lung biopsy (histopathology) – fibrinous obliteration of the lumen of the respiratory and membranous bronchioles.

Grading

NIH proposed scoring system

- Score 0: No symptoms of FEV1> 80% or LFS = 2
- Score 1: Mild symptoms or FEV1 60% to 79% or LFS = 3 to 5
- Score 2: Moderate symptoms or FEV1 40% to 59% or LFS 6 to 9
- Score 3: Severe symptoms or FEV1 ≤39% or LFS = 10 to 12

LFS is the global assessment of lung function after the diagnosis of bronchiolitis obliterans (BO) has already been established. See organ-scoring NIH proposed definition and organ scoring system in Chapter 13, chronic GVHD, scoring/grading.

Grading of BO among patients receiving lung grafts

- Mild: (FEV1 66% to 80%)
- Moderate: (FEV1 51% to 65%)
- Severe: (FEV1 <50%)

Risk Factors

Allogeneic transplantation – BO is rare in autologous HSCT. It usually occurs in association with cGVHD and hypogammaglobulinemia. The risk increases with age and with prior abnormalities of pulmonary function.

Treatment

Corticosteroids in combination with calcineurin inhibitors may stabilize PFTs. Monitor IgG levels and replete when IgG levels are less than 400 (cutoff levels may vary by institution). Some centers have reported stabilization or improvement on extracorporeal photopheresis.

Recently azithromycin has been suggested as a possible treatment but there is little data, and clinical trials are needed to support this approach.[1]

Bronchiolitis Obliterans–Organizing Pneumonia

Diagnosis

- fever, dyspnea, and cough
- Crackles more than wheezes
- CXR abnormal
- PFTs with restrictive pattern
- reduced DLCO and lung volumes
- Associated with acute and chronic GVHD. This should be distinguished from bronchiolitis obliterans without organizing pneumonia.

Treatment

Most patients respond to glucocorticosteroids 1 to 2 mg/kg daily. Often treatment must be given for 6 months or more. It is managed identically to BOOP occurring outside the transplantation setting.

Pulmonary Veno-occlusive Disease

Pulmonary veno-occlusive disease is a rare complication after HSCT. Patients may present with dyspnea, normal pulmonary function tests, and no evidence of infection.

Diagnosis

Right-sided cardiac catheterization is required to document the presence of pulmonary hypertension (without emboli). Lung biopsy should confirm the diagnosis.

SUGGESTED READINGS

Chien JW, Martin PJ, Gooley TA, et al. Airflow obstruction after myeloablative allogeneic hematopoietic stem cell transplantation. *Am J Respir Crit Care Med.* 2003;168:208–214.

Afessa B, Litzow MR, Tefferi A. Bronchiolitis obliterans and other late onset non-infectious pulmonary complications in hematopoietic stem cell transplantation (Review). *Bone Marrow Transplant.* 2001;28:425–434.

REFERENCE

1. Khalid M, Al Saghir A, Saleemi S, et al. Azithromycin in bronchiolitis obliterans complicating bone marrow transplantation: A preliminary study. *Eur Resp J.* 2005;25:490–493.

19. VENO-OCCLUSIVE DISEASE

Hepatic Veno-occlusive disease (VOD) (sometimes referred to as sinusoidal obstruction syndrome [SOS]) is a process of central venular occlusion characterized by sinusoidal endothelial injury, subendothelial edema, intrahepatic obstruction of blood flow, hepatocellular necrosis, and intense fibrosis. Its pathophysiology is complex but reflects a cascade of drug toxicity, cytokine injury, and hypoxic, free radical-mediated damage to Zone 3 of the hepatic acinus. It occurs in 5% to 20% of patients and ranges from a mild self-limiting illness to a severe disease with almost universal fatality. It generally occurs early after conditioning, that is, day 0 to 30 (although later onset can occur).

RISK FACTORS

It is important to try to identify patients at high risk for VOD early. In doing so, preventative measures (such as reducing sinusoidal toxins) can be implemented.

- Multiple alkylating agents in conditioning regimen (especially cyclophosphamide, busulfan, and BCNU), total body irradiation (TBI), liver disease pre transplant (as reflected increased SGOT), second or greater transplant, allogeneic donor (significantly less common after auto HSCT and after T-cell–depleted allogeneic HSCT, Mylotarg exposure (especially if within 3 to 4 months of HSCT).
- Sirolimus in association with high-dose regimens, particular busulfan.
- Other associations include high-dose IVIG use, recurrent febrile episodes, estrogen administration and prior viral hepatitis, nonalcoholic steatohepatitis, previous transplantation (as mentioned earlier), iron overload, and liver involvement with tumor.

CLINICAL MANIFESTATIONS

- Abdominal pain, particularly right upper quadrant (RUQ).

- Increasing ascites and peripheral edema with associated weight gain.
- Unexplained increase in drug levels (e.g., cyclosporine or tacrolimus).

DIAGNOSIS

- A triad of clinical symptoms and signs with two or more of the following:
    - Weight gain (>5% above baseline), ascites, fluid retention ascites and fluid avidity is due to portal hypertension and hepatorenal syndrome, with low fractional excretion of sodium (FENa).
    - RUQ pain/hepatomegaly
- Hyperbilirubinemia (Bilirubin >2 mg/dL)

- Baltimore criteria >5%; Seattle criteria >2%, with the latter being less-specific.
- Ultrasound with Doppler is helpful to look for reversal of portal flow, to document ascites and rule out cholangitis.
- Computerized tomography (CT) and magnetic resonance imaging (MRI) should be ordered as indicated to rule out other causes of liver disease.
- Liver biopsy and wedged hepatic venous pressure gradient assessment can be very helpful but are potentially risky in coagulopathic patients. Biopsy should be done only via the transvenous route. Before biopsy, correct coagulopathy (factor VII concentrates can be helpful and it is important to keep platelets greater than 30,000/μL if procedure done). Biopsy is the gold standard if there is diagnostic uncertainty.

MAJOR DIFFERENTIAL DIAGNOSIS

- Graft-versus-host disease of liver; cyclosporine toxicity, estrogen therapy, drug toxicity (e.g., MTX, cyclosporine, azole antifungals), hyperalimentation, infection (sepsis, cholangitis lenta), viral hepatitis (Figure 19.1).

HALLMARKS OF SEVERE/FATAL DISEASE

- Multiorgan failure (MOF – defined as one or more of the following: creatinine $2\times$ to $3\times$ or greater, above baseline, O_2 sat <90% on room air, encephalopathy).

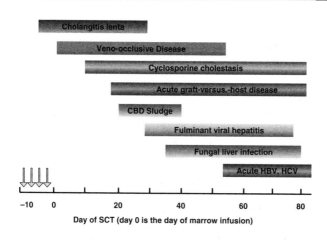

Figure 19.1 Veno-Occlussive Disease

CBD, common bile duct; CHF, congestive heart failure; EBV, *Epstein-Barr virus*; GVHD, graft-versus-host disease; HBV, *Hepatitis B virus*; HCV, *Hepatitis C virus*; SCT, stem cell trnsplantation; VOD, veno-occlusive disease.

- Presence of ascites, rapid weight gain, and rapid rise of bilirubin.
- Prognosis of severe disease is poor (Day +100 mortality >90%) if present.

PROPHYLAXIS

- Ursodiol – the benefit observed to date is marginal.
- Defibrotide is showing promise and is now under study in both Europe and the United States for this indication.[1,2]

TREATMENT

- Supportive care, analgesia as needed.
- Use of diuretics can be helpful. It is prudent to avoid aggressive use of diuretics until fluid overload is significantly symptomatic since they are likely to result in volume depletion and hepatorenal syndrome.
- Transfusion to keep HCT >30 to 35 to maintain renal blood flow is the most useful strategy.
- Pay careful attention to bleeding (factor deficiency and platelet refractoriness characteristic).
- Minimize nephrotoxins and hepatotoxins (e.g., adjust tacrolimus, cyclosporine, or sirolimus).
- TPA/and heparin are not recommended.[3]
- Defibrotide is an investigational agent currently considered the most promising treatment to date. Clinical trials in the United States and Europe show response rates of 36% to 50% for established severe VOD with D +100 survival of 40% to 50% (vs <10% expected).[4,5,6]
- Infections can be a major problem in VOD. It is important to consider spontaneous bacterial peritonitis (SBP) and be aware that patients may not be overtly febrile. A low threshold for antibiotics and broad coverage is recommended.

REFERENCES

1. Chalandon Y, Roosnek E, Mermillod B, et al. Prevention of veno-occlusive disease with defibrotide after allogeneic stem cell transplantation. *Biol Blood Marrow Transplant.* 2004 May;10(5):347–354.
2. Corbacioglu S, Hönig M, Lahr G, et al. Stem cell transplantation in children with infantile osteopetrosis is associated with a high incidence of VOD, which could be prevented with defibrotide. *Bone Marrow Transplant.* 2006 Oct;38(8):547–553. Epub 2006 Sep 4.
3. Bearman SI, Lee JL, Barón AE, McDonald GB. Treatment of hepatic venocclusive disease with recombinant human tissue plasminogen activator and heparin in 42 marrow transplant patients. *Blood.* 1997 Mar 1;89(5):1501–1506.
4. Richardson PG, Elias AD, Krishnan A, et al. Treatment of severe veno-occlusive disease with defibrotide: Compassionate use

results in response without significant toxicity in a high-risk population. *Blood.* 1998 Aug 1;92(3):737–744.

5. Richardson PG, Murakami C, Jin Z, Warren D, et al. Multi-institutional use of defibrotide in 88 patients after stem cell transplantation with severe veno-occlusive disease and multisystem organ failure: Response without significant toxicity in a high-risk population and factors predictive of outcome. *Blood.* 2002 Dec 15;100(13):4337–4343. Epub 2002 Aug 1.

6. Chopra R, Eaton JD, Grassi A, Potter M, et al. Defibrotide for the treatment of hepatic veno-occlusive disease: Results of the European compassionate-use study. *Br J Haematol.* 2000 Dec;111(4):1122–1129.

20. SPECIAL TRANSFUSION-RELATED SITUATIONS

A complete discussion of transfusion reactions is beyond the scope of this manual. The incidence of infection through a blood transfusion has been greatly reduced, given the improvements in donor screening and processing techniques. The most significant infectious risk of transfusions is due to bacterially contaminated platelets. Platelets must be stored at room temperature and on an average 1 in 3,000 bags are contaminated with bacteria proven by culture. The risk of an infection through a platelet transfusion is approximately 1 in 20,000.

TRANSFUSION-RELATED ACUTE LUNG INJURY

Mechanism

The risk of transfusion-related acute lung injury (TRALI) is estimated at 1 case per 5,000 transfusions. It is characterized by acute onset of hypoxemia and the appearance of bilateral infiltration on chest X-ray within 6 hours of transfusion of a plasma-containing product. The exact mechanism is unknown but in a subset of patients, donor antibodies (usually antiHLA) react with the recipient's white blood cells resulting in both release of intracellular inflammatory mediators and leukoagglutination in the lungs.

Differential Diagnosis

It may be difficult to distinguish TRALI from circulatory overload or adult respiratory distress syndrome.

Therapy

Care is supportive including supplemental oxygen. Approximately 75% of patients will require mechanical ventilation. Most patients will recover in 2 to 4 days; mortality rate is 5% to 10%.

RED CELL APLASIA

Mechanism

Preformed antibody present in the recipient is capable of causing hemolysis and preventing recovery of red blood cell production. This is most common when the recipient is of type O and the donor is of type A, but it can occur whenever the recipient has preexistent antibody. This problem is also more prevalent in reduced-intensity transplantation, where it may take longer for B cells that produce the antibodies to be eradicated. It manifests as continued transfusion requirements despite full engraftment.

Differential Diagnosis

It must be distinguished from failure of erythropoietin production and hemolytic anemia. The two effects are easily distinguished:

- Check the reticulocyte count. This is the best measure of active red blood cell (RBC) production. If it is elevated, there is no deficiency of erythropoietin.
- Erythropoietin level can also be checked. Erythropoietin levels vary with the degree of anemia. If the hemoglobin (Hb) level is normal, the erythropoietin level will be low. However, a low erythropoietin level in a patient with anemia suggests failure of erythropoietin production .
- Check an isohemagglutinin titer. If the titer is low, for example, 1:2 or 1:4, it will usually decline with time. If it is high, it may require therapy.

Therapy

- Folate replacement.
- If the titer is high or persists, alternatives include plasmapheresis and rituximab therapy. The isohemagglutinin titer and reticulocyte count can be measured to assess response to therapy.

TRANSFUSION–ASSOCIATED GRAFT-VERSUS-HOST DISEASE

Mechanism

Transfusion–associated graft-versus-host disease (TA-GVHD) is a rare but a devastating and fatal complication of blood transfusions that affect primarily immunocompromised recipients. It is not usually seen after HSCT since the donor lymphocytes and donor hematopoiesis are genetically the same. It is occasionally observed after organ transplantation where viable lymphocytes in the organ are passively transferred to the recipient. Since most organ transplantation involves significant histocompatibility differences, these viable lymphocytes may proliferate and induce GVHD. In contrast to the hematopoietic stem cell transplantation setting, the lymphocytes also attack normal recipient hematopoiesis, resulting in marrow failure. The other setting in which this can occur is when viable lymphocytes are transfused into patients who cannot reject them. Most commonly this results from transfusion of nonirradiated or non–leukocyte-depleted blood products into immunocompromised recipients. However, it can rarely occur with family member-directed donor transfusion, where the donor is homozygous and the recipient is heterozygous. In this setting, the non-immunocompromised recipient cannot clear the transfused T cells. The transfused T cells induce GVHD and marrow failure by the mechanism detailed earlier.

Differential Diagnosis

Some severe viral infections (e.g., CMV, perhaps HHV-6) can give rise to clinical syndromes that mimic TA-GVHD. Diagnosis is confirmed by identifying donor T cells by human leukocyte antigen (HLA) typing or chimerism analysis.

Therapy

Outcomes are usually poor. Therapy for acute GVHD is appropriate but if hematopoiesis has been destroyed, a reduced-intensity transplant from a histocompatible donor may be needed to restore stem cell function.

21. CARDIOVASCULAR COMPLICATIONS

MYOPERICARDITIS

Cyclophosphamide cardiotoxicity is idiosyncratic and independent of baseline cardiac function. When used in high doses, cyclophosphamide can induce myopericarditis that can be associated with pericardial tamponade or pulseless electrical activity (PEA) arrest and death. Milder forms may lead to congestive heart failure, requiring appropriate therapy. More common is the development of myocardial edema that can result in reduction in electrocardiogram (ECG) voltage but no functional consequences.

Clinical Manifestations

- Shortness of breath, chest discomfort (often pleuritic and improved with sitting up), cough, fever, tachycardia.

Diagnosis

- Pericardial rub, ST segment elevation, PR depression.
- Echocardiogram may show fluid; with impending tamponade, may also have diastolic indentation or collapse of the right ventricle. Aspiration under fluoroscopic guidance may be required for presumed infectious or malignant etiologies.

Treatment

- If manifestations are mild, supportive care is usually adequate.
- Nonsteroidal anti-inflammatory drugs (NSAIDS) are not used in patients with thrombocytopenia.
- If cyclophosphamide is the presumed etiology, there is no specific therapy.
- If the underlying problem is infectious or malignant it is treated specifically.
- Pericardiocentesis or a pericardial window if tamponade develops.

ARRHYTHMIAS AND CONDUCTION ABNORMALITIES

Arrhythmias are uncommon during hematopoietic stem cell transplantation (HSCT) except as reflections of preexistent heart disease. New onset rhythm disturbances or conduction delay may be due to dimethyl sulfoxide (DMSO) at the time of stem cell infusion, cyclophosphamide, volume overload, infection, medications, infarction, cardiomyopathy, pulmonary embolus, electrolyte abnormalities, and thyroid disease. DMSO has been associated with heart block and fluctuations in blood pressure.

Diagnosis

■ Complete electrolyte evaluation, thyroid-stimulating hormone (TSH), ECG, chest X-ray (CXR), and echocardiogram when indicated.

Treatment

■ If DMSO is implicated, slow the rate of infusion, hydrate, and observe. It is rare that an intervention is required. If severe, hydrocortisone may be given in addition to diphenhydramine. See DMSO toxicity in Chapter 7, Stem Cell Infusion.

HYPERTENSIVE CRISIS

Hypertensive crisis occurs most commonly in patients with underlying hypertension, but it clearly can be related to the use of calcineurin inhibitors (cyclosporine, tacrolimus). This is treated with calcium-channel blockers, angiotensin-converting enzyme (ACE) inhibitors (if renal function is satisfactory), β-blockers, and in severe cases, with nitroprusside or intravenous nitroglycerine. There is a risk of posterior encephalopathy and cortical blindness. Rarely, the calcineurin inhibitor must be stopped and it may be replaced with mycophenolate mofetil or sirolimus without fear of exacerbating the hypertension. Hypertension should be well controlled in patients with thrombocytopenia.

PATENT FORMEN OVALE

Approximately 10% of the population has a patent foramen ovale. This is generally not of physiologic concern; however, this may pose a problem during the infusion of stem cells, particularly if a filter is not used. This may result in cerebral emboli due to cell aggregates in the product. We recommend using a standard blood filter for all stem cell products that may have cellular or fibrin aggregates.

22. NEUROLOGIC COMPLICATIONS

Neurologic toxicity is common and often multifactorial. The primary causes of neurologic injury are (1) drug toxicity, (2) infection, (3) toxic metabolic encephalopathy, and (4) hemorrhage. It is convenient to consider neurologic injury occurring early after transplantation and that occurring late after transplantation separately. Early toxicity tends to be related to immediate problems with conditioning regimen effects. Preexistent neurological problems related to malignancy or metabolic encephalopathy are likely to increase the risk of immediate posttransplantation neurologic symptoms. Later events are often related to prolonged immunoincompetence and the effects of calcineurin inhibitors.

EARLY-POSTTRANSPLANT PERIOD

Calcineurin Inhibitors

- The calcineurin inhibitors (CNI) cyclosporine and tacrolimus are probably the single most frequent cause of neurologic toxicity. The most common manifestations are tremor and burning palmar and plantar dysesthesias. However, headache, depression, confusion, somnolence, and nystagmus may be observed. Seizures may occur, especially in association with hypomagnesemia, hypertension, hypocholesterolemia, infections, and high blood levels of CNI.

- A unique complication of CNIs is cortical blindness and posterior leukoencephalopathy. This syndrome is often observed in association with the new onset of hypertension, suggesting that there is cerebral edema due to abnormalities of pressure regulation in the posterior circulation. Many of the radiologic manifestations are similar to those seen in hypertensive encephalopathy. The most common pattern is white matter edema in the posterior circulation. It may or may not persist despite continued use of the drug. Although there are reports to the contrary, most clinicians believe that cyclosporine and tacrolimus are cross-reactive; therefore, substitution of one for the other may not be useful. Newer agents such as sirolimus or mycophenolate mofetil have no known neurological toxicity and may be appropriate substitutes for CNI. Establishing a successful immunosuppressive regimen in this setting can be quite difficult and may require persistent use of the offending agent with an effort to maintain excellent blood pressure control.

■ A frequent complication of the use of CNI is the development of thrombotic microangiopathy. These microangiopathies are associated with evidence of hemolysis; typically, schistocytes are observed in the blood smear and there is a reduction in haptoglobin. Because of the renal vascular involvement, hypertension and azotemia are generally concomitantly observed.

■ Other less common manifestations of these agents include coma, optic disc edema, aphasia, paralysis, insomnia, somnolence, and rigidity.

Supportive Medications

■ The use of narcotics, benzodiazepines, antihistamines, and antiemetics, often in combination, are probably the most frequent cause of altered mental status or seizures.

■ Careful attention to polypharmacy will help prevent complications related to these agents.

Infections

■ The most frequent central nervous system (CNS) infections are due to reactivation of toxoplasmosis and fungal infections, most commonly the Aspergillus species. Angioinvasive molds such as *Aspergillus* and *Mucor* may spread to the brain via hematogenous routes or by direct invasion from the sinuses. *Cryptococcus* is less common.

■ *Human herpes virus*-6 (HHV-6) infections are increasingly recognized after transplantation. Neurological involvement is typically in the temporal lobes, and the diagnosis may be made by identifying HHV-6 by polymerase chain reaction on spinal fluid.[1]

■ Reactivation of herpes viruses such as *Herpes simplex* and *Varicella zoster* are usually prevented with prophylactic acyclovir, but resistant strains may be encountered.

■ Less commonly, *JC* virus may result in progressive multifocal encephalopathy.

■ Rarely, West Nile virus and other Arboviruses can be a problem in the appropriate season.

Conditioning Regimen Toxicity

■ Busulfan, in the doses used in stem cell transplantation, results in generalized seizures in approximately 5% of patients unless they receive prophylactic anticonvulsants.

■ Total body irradiation does not appear to have intrinsic brain toxicity; however, in patients with prior mediastinal irradiation, it must be avoided or spinal cord tolerance may be exceeded and cord transections can occur.

■ Alemtuzumab (Campath) in combination with chemotherapeutic agents has been suggested to have a high incidence of progressive sensorimotor neuropathy and myelitis, although this effect seems to be associated with the high risk of viral reactivation that is associated with this agent.

■ High-dose cyclophosphamide can cause the syndrome of inappropriate antidiuretic hormone (SIADH) secretion, presumably via a central mechanism. Rarely, if incorrectly treated, this can result in central pontine myelinolysis.

Malignancy

■ Leukemic or lymphomatous meningitis that occurs before the transplantation increases the risk of both relapse after the transplantation and the risk of nonspecific injury such as leukoencephalopathy.

Therapy

■ Treatment of neurologic complications requires establishment of the correct diagnosis and specific management.

■ Treatment of the seizures requires recognition that cyclosporine and tacrolimus levels may be altered by anticonvulsants. For instance, phenobarbital induces cytochrome P450 to the degree that massive doses of CNI may be required to maintain adequate levels. Furthermore, there is reluctance to use carbamazepine, phenytoin, and some of the other anticonvulsants, because of concerns about their effects on the incipient marrow recovery. Levetiracetam

(Keppra), benzodiazepines, and gabapentin may be more useful because of their limited drug interactions and low risk of marrow toxicity.

LATE-POSTTRANSPLANT PERIOD

■ Once the graft is functioning acceptably and the patient has recovered, the causes of neurologic injury shift. The major risks in this period are the manifestations of opportunistic infections and the long-term toxicity of strategies used to prevent or control rejection and graft-versus-host disease (GVHD). Viral meningoencephalitis may occur with most of the herpes virus family, especially Cytomegalovirus, *Varicella zoster* virus, HHV-6, and *Herpes simplex*. Early diagnosis and aggressive appropriate antiviral therapy such as acyclovir, ganciclovir, or foscarnet is often effective and can result in complete resolution of the infection. *Varicella zoster* virus reactivation can result not only in the well-known cutaneous manifestations but also (especially in severely immunocompromised patients) in severe abdominal pain without dermatomal vesicles. High-dose acyclovir can itself result in a reversible encephalopathy in susceptible patients. Postherpetic neuralgia is occasionally observed and may be ameliorated with agents such as amitriptyline and gabapentin. *Epstein-Barr* virus may be reactivate and result in lymphoproliferative disorders that have a predilection to extranodal dissemination, including the brain.

■ CNS toxoplasmosis typically occurs in the 6 months following the transplantation, but it can occur as a later manifestation as well. Trimethoprim/sulfamethoxazole used for pneumocystis prophylaxis will often prevent CNS toxoplasmosis as well. Computerized tomography scan and magnetic resonance imaging usually show the typically ring-enhancing lesions when the infection occurs late, in contrast to the less definitive appearance of these scans in the early-posttransplant period.

■ Progressive multifocal encephalopathy is occasionally encountered, however, it is rare. Some reports have demonstrated improvement with purine analog therapy, but there is no consistently-valuable therapy for this disease.

Neuromuscular and Peripheral Nerve Complications

■ The most bothersome long-term CNS toxicity is a coarse tremor related to calcineurin inhibitors. This resolves when the drugs are stopped.

■ Steroid myopathies are often quite debilitating. Efforts to improve muscle strength involve using supplemental immunosuppressants to allow dose reductions in corticosteroids. Mycophenolate mofetil appears to be a useful agent in this regard.

■ Muscle spasms are a particular aggravation for many patients after allogeneic stem cell grafting. These can occur in almost any muscles, although the lower extremities and hands are the most common. The spasms may or may not be painful, and they are often triggered by muscular activity such as writing or typing. While CNI are implicated in the development of this problem, many patients will continue to have such spasms long after CNI have been stopped. Typically, therapeutic trials with quinine, baclofen, valium, high dose vitamin E, magnesium replacement, and potassium replacement are tried. Some manipulations seem to work for some people, but there is no consistently useful approach.

■ Guillain-Barre syndrome has been reported at increased frequency after allogeneic stem cell transplantation. Guillain-Barre syndrome usually responds to standard treatments.

■ Myasthenia gravis appears primarily to be a complication of chronic GVHD, and it may respond to immunosuppression, plasmapheresis, and anticholinesterase therapy.

■ There are rare cases of focal demyelination of the CNS that look similar to multiple sclerosis. It has been suggested that this is a manifestation of GVHD, although there is little objective support for that contention.

REFERENCE

1. Seeley WW, Marty FM, Holmes TM, et al. Post-transplant acute limbic encephalitis: an HHV6-induced neurological syndrome? *Neurology.* 2007;69:156–165.

23. CYSTITIS

There are two main causes of hemorrhagic cystitis in the transplant patient: conditioning regimen–related toxicity and viral infection. Cystitis that occurs early (day 1 to 14) is usually caused by the conditioning agents, and is usually related to high-dose cyclophosphamide. The incidence of early cystitis reduced with the use of aggressive hydration with forced saline diuresis or the use of Mesna for uroprotection. Mesna binds to an inactive metabolite of cyclophosphamide, acrolein, preventing urothelial inflammation. Mesna is effective only during cyclophosphamide metabolism/excretion and not once hemorrhagic cystitis is established. We recommend prehydration with 1,000 cc of D5NS with 20 mEq/L of KCl at 500 cc/hr for at least 2 hours precyclophosphamide dose and maintenance of hydration with D5½NS at 200 cc/hr for 12 hours after cyclophosphamide using furosemide if necessary to keep urine output >200 cc/hr.

Hemorrhagic cystitis that occurs after day 14 is usually due to a viral infection. The two most common infections include BK virus and Adenovirus infection.

DIAGNOSIS

Urine should be sent for urinalysis, bacterial and viral culture, and BK and Adenovirus polymerase chain reaction (PCR). If adenovirus infection is confirmed it is important to monitor for systemic disease and treat if it disseminates.

TREATMENT

There is no defined treatment for BK-associated cystitis and no treatment can be recommended at this time. There are anecdotal reports of using quinolones, cidofovir, and leflunomide for treatment, but in most cases cystitis resolves spontaneously and requires only supportive/symptomatic treatment.

Mild Cystitis

Pain control, hydration, and bladder antispasmodics. Phenazopryidine 200 mg orally TID should be used for burning discomfort.

Maximum use is for 3 days; use for more than 3 days increases the risk of methemoglobinemia.

Severe Cystitis with Bleeding

- Keep platelets above 30,000 to 50,000.
- Monitor coagulation studies.
- Three-way bladder irrigation is indicated for clots (especially if obstruction develops) or a decrease in urine output.
- Antispasmodics – flavoxate 100 to 200 mg orally 3 to 4 times/ day (used for both pain and spasm).
- Hyosciamine can also help.
- Oxybutynin (Oxytrol) 1 patch (3.9 mg/day) applied twice weekly (every 3 to 4 days).
- Tolterodine 1 to 2 mg PO BID. Use with caution, since it is metabolized by the P450 system and will interact with calcineurin inhibitors and azoles.

24. DONOR LYMPHOCYTE INFUSION

Donor lymphocyte infusion (DLI) is an effective method to induce graft-versus-leukemia (GVL) and is commonly used to treat patients with hematologic malignancies who have relapsed after allogeneic stem cell transplantation or to treat patients with falling donor chimerism after reduced-intensity conditioning. Previous reviews from Europe and North America have reported complete hematologic and cytogenetic response rates in over 75% of patients with stable phase chronic myelogenous leukemia (CML) treated with DLI following hematopoietic stem cell transplantation, although outcomes are significantly worse in other hematologic malignancies.

INDUCTION OF GRAFT-VERSUS-LEUKEMIA

- In patients who need DLI while still on immunosuppression, a rapid taper of immunosuppressants will often result in a graft-versus-host disease (GVHD) flare that can induce a remission or full chimerism.
- In patients who are off all immunosuppression, DLI is a reasonable strategy to induce GVL.

COLLECTION AND ADMINISTRATION OF DONOR LYMPHOCYTE INFUSION

- Lymphocytes are typically collected without filgrastim stimulation.
- Cells can be used fresh; however, it is useful to cryopreserve cells in aliquots of 1 to 5×10^7 CD3$^+$ cells/kg body weight.
- For indolent diseases, administration of cells in gradually increasing numbers separated by 4 to 8 weeks will reduce the risk of GVHD. For instance, start with 1×10^7 CD3$^+$ cells/kg. If there is no GVHD and the desired response has not been achieved by 6 weeks increase the dose to 5×10^7 CD3$^+$ cells/kg. Doses beyond 10^8 CD3$^+$ cells/kg are usually not desirable.
- For aggressive diseases, typical doses of 10^8 CD3$^+$ cells/kg are administered as a single dose.

- DLI usually can be administered in the outpatient area. Normal procedures for blood product administration are followed.
- It takes several weeks to observe GVHD and/or GVL.

THREE IMPORTANT COMPLICATIONS OF DLI

- The development of GVHD is a major complication of DLI. The incidence of acute GVHD grades II to IV after DLI ranges from 45% to 80% in large studies.[1,2] Although the development of GVHD has correlated with clinical antileukemic effect after DLI, there have been patients who have experienced complete responses in the absence of clinical GVHD. Methods to reduce GVHD after DLI include the infusion of low numbers of donor cells or infusion of selected lymphocyte cell populations. Patients with active acute overall GVHD grade II or greater or extensive chronic GVHD requiring systemic immune suppressive medications are ineligible to receive DLI.
- The second important complication of DLI is marrow aplasia. The etiology of this complication is unclear, but may represent a form of graft-versus-hematopoiesis or another immunologic phenomenon. Usually, this marrow aplasia is temporary, but the use of cytokine therapy may expedite marrow recovery. Rarely, administration of marrow or peripheral blood stem cells from the donor is required. If there is active GVHD, depletion of T cells from the product should be considered.
- Finally, transfusion reactions can occur during DLI. These are managed as any other transfusion reaction is managed.

REFERENCES

1. Schmid C, Labopin M, Nagler A, et al. Donor lymphocyte infusion in the treatment of first hematological relapse after allogeneic stem-cell transplantation in adults with acute myeloid leukemia: a retrospective risk factors analysis and comparison with other strategies by the EBMT Acute Leukemia Working Party. *J Clin Oncol.* 2007 Nov 1;25(31):4938–4945. Epub 2007 Oct 1.

2. Collins RH Jr, Goldstein S, Giralt S, et al. Donor leukocyte infusions in acute lymphocytic leukemia. *Bone Marrow Transplant.* 2000 Sep;26(5):511–516.

25. TRANSPLANTATION: REGULATION AND ACCREDITATION

Governmental regulations exist at both the federal and the state level. At the federal level, the U.S. Food and Drug Administration (FDA) is responsible for enforcing the regulations for human cells, tissues, and cellular- and tissue-based products. Cellular products are regulated either under cGTP 21CFR 1271, cGMP 21 CFR 210, or in part under the device regulations. Cell therapy products that are more than minimally manipulated (including all gene therapy products) most often need an FDA IND exemption and at least Institutional Review Board (IRB) approval before use. Some states have developed licensure processes, certificate programs, and so on, but other states have few specific regulations.

There are three voluntary professional organizations that set standards and accredit various components of hematopoietic stem cell transplantation (HSCT). The three foundations are Foundation for the Accreditation of Cellular Therapy (FACT), The American Association of Blood Banks (AABB), and the National Marrow Donor Program (NMDP).

Foundation for the Accreditation of Cellular Therapy is a partnership between two organizations, one that is based on clinical outcome and the other that is laboratory based. Combined, they provide minimal guidelines and standards to all sources and phases for facilities and individuals who perform HSCT. It is important to know your program's specific regulations under FDA, state, and other voluntary accredited programs.

Appendix

BODY SURFACE AREA (BSA)

$$\sqrt{\frac{\text{height (cm)} \times \text{weight (kg)}}{3{,}600}}$$

1.1 Ideal Body Weight Formula (IBW)
Male IBW = 50 kg + (2.3 kg × actual height in inches – 60)
Female IBW = 45 kg + (2.3 kg × actual height in inches – 60)
1.2 Adjusted Ideal Body Weight = (Actual body weight – Ideal weight) 0.4 + Ideal weight

Some protocols use charts, wrist size, body frame, and so on to determine ideal weight. And some even modify the adjusted weight.

ECOG/ZUBBROD PERFORMANCE STATUS

0	Fully active, able to carry on all pre-disease performance without restriction
1	Restricted in physically strenuous activity but ambulatory and able to carry out work of a light or sedentary nature, e.g. light house work, office work
2	Ambulatory and capable of all selfcare but unable to carry out any work activities. Up and about more than 50% of waking hours
3	Capable of only limited selfcare, confined to bed or chair more than 50% of waking hours
4	Completely disabled. Cannot carry on any selfcare. Totally confined to bed or chair
5	Dead

Karnofsky Performance Scale

100 Normal, no complaints, no evidence of disease.
 90 Able to carry on normal activity: minor symptoms of disease.
 80 Normal activity with effort: some symptoms of disease.

70 Cares for self: unable to carry on normal activity or active work.

60 Requires occasional assistance but is able to care for needs.

50 Requires considerable assistance and frequent medical care.

40 Disabled: requires special care and assistance.

30 Severely disabled: hospitalization is indicated, death not imminent.

20 Very sick, hospitalization necessary: active treatment necessary.

10 Moribund, fatal processes progressing rapidly.

0 Dead

Index

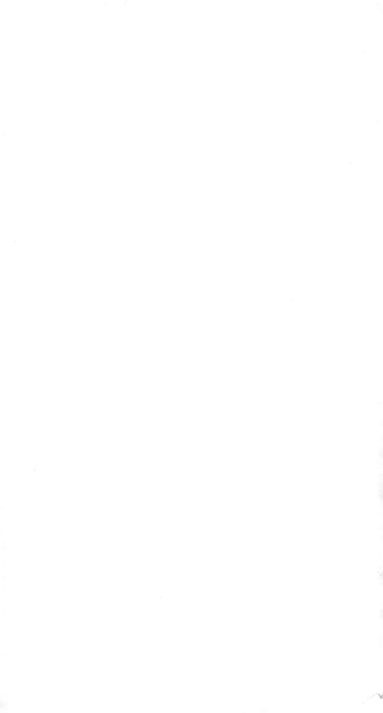